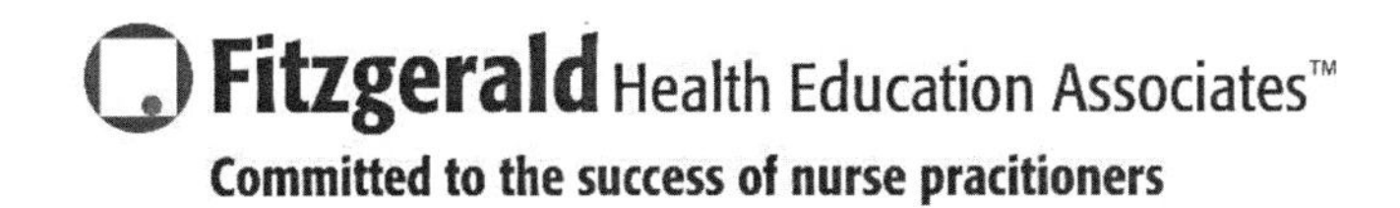

Cue Card Series

Pediatric Physical Assessment

Tenth Edition

Susan Feeney, DNP, FNP-BC, NP-C

Margaret A. Fitzgerald,
DNP, FNP-BC, NP-C, FAANP, CSP, FAAN, DC

Fitzgerald Health Education Associates, LLC
85 Flagship Drive
North Andover, Massachusetts 01845-6154
(978) 794-8366 · FAX (978) 794-2455
Email: cs@fhea.com Website: fhea.com

ISBN 978-1-57942604-0

Tenth Edition

Last digit indicates print number: 10 9 8 7 6 5 4 3 2 1

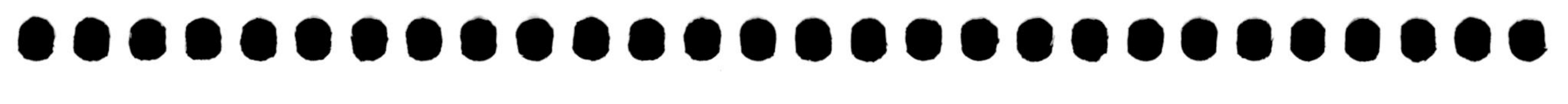

Fitzgerald Health Education Associates, LLC
North Andover, Massachusetts

STATEMENT OF LIABILITY

The information contained in this work has been thoroughly researched and checked for accuracy. However, clinical practice is a dynamic process and new information becomes available daily. Prudent practice dictates that the clinician consult further sources prior to applying information from this book. Fitzgerald Health Education Associates, LLC disclaims any liability, loss, injury, or damage incurred as a consequence, directly or indirectly, from the use and application of any of the contents of this volume.

Acknowledgments

I would like to thank Margaret Fitzgerald for offering me the opportunity to work with so many new and experienced NPs and for being such a wonderful mentor and generous colleague. I would like to thank my colleague and dear friend Wendy Wright who believed in me and has supported me from the moment we met. Finally I would like to thank my husband Brian and our daughters, Allison and Kaitlin for their unwavering love and support. I am truly blessed.

Editors' Note

Our thanks to Anita Hunter, PhD, CNS, CPNP, FAAN, the author of the first five editions of this work and Michelle A. Beauchesne, DNSc, CPNP, FNAP, FAANP for her contributions to the sixth and seventh editions. Their contributions to the NP profession have been numerous and we are grateful for their collaboration with Fitzgerald Health Education Associates over the years.

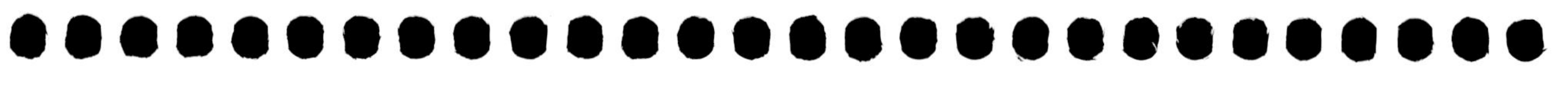

Foreword

The most important steps in properly assessing a patient's health problem are an accurate and thorough health history, followed by the appropriate physical exam. The Cue Card series is designed to do just that, by providing a step-by-step guide through the pediatric health history and physical examination. Included in this concise guide are cues for common variations from the norm as well as suggestions for the documentation of your findings.

The Cue Card series is an excellent resource for any healthcare provider, whether student or seasoned clinician, who wants to hone clinical skills. Watch for additional titles in this series.

Margaret A. Fitzgerald, DNP, FNP-BC, NP-C, FAANP, CSP, FAAN, DCC, FNAP

President and Principal Lecturer Fitzgerald Health Education Associates, North Andover, MA

About the format of the Cue Cards:

Content is organized into general information and age specific categories.

Procedures, directives to the clinician, or actions which the patient must perform appear in italics in the same manner as this sentence.

Text that appears without emphasis is suitable for dictating the findings from the physical exam.

> Abnormalities and "heads up" for special situations are boxed and shaded in the same manner as this paragraph. The list is not intended to be exhaustive but to include many of the abnormalities commonly seen in a primary care setting.

FIRST:

Remember children live and grow within the context of family, peers, school, and the broader environment. In recent years there have been many changing variations in the family unit. The role of the healthcare provider is to partner with families and build on their strengths to help provide the optimal environment for children to grow and develop.

SECOND:

Each child understands the world differently and at his or her own pace, although the pattern of development is fixed and predictable. A child's culture and ethnicity along with intellectual, emotional, and social development defines his or her world view, sense of reality, relationship to others, and perceptions of health and illness.

THIRD:

Individual differences among children are normal and represent developmental variations. Children are generally healthy and have many adaptive capabilities, which increase their resilience in the face of limitations.

FINALLY:

Remember thoroughness is the cornerstone of assessment at any age. Observe, listen, and document carefully and systematically. Approach every child and family with empathy and respect.

Pediatric Health History
Table of Contents

Pediatric Physical Assessment

Table of Contents

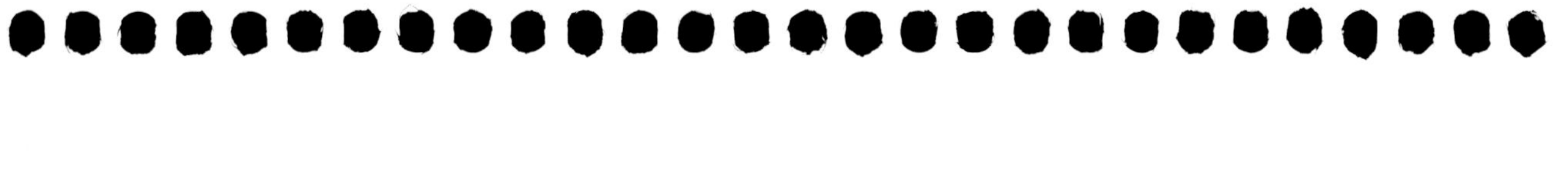

Cue Card Series

Pediatric Health History

I. General Data

Applies to all children ages birth to adolescent

Risk assessment:

A comprehensive health history with particular attention to ***known risk factors is an integral part of any developmental assessment.*** *Obtain as much of this information as is appropriate, given time and reason for visit, prior to conducting the physical exam. Some of this information can be completed via a preformed questionnaire, one-to-one interview, telephone interview or a combination of the three. This information can help identify actual or potential problems for the child and/or the family.*

A comprehensive ***Family History*** *helps identify known genetic conditions as well as familial predisposition for illnesses.*

Draw a genogram, which is a simplified diagram of a *family's genealogy that shows at least 3 generations of family members and their relationships to each other. Identify known illnesses, health conditions and behaviors*. Available at www.hhs.gov/familyhistory

Use of genogram helps identify known genetic conditions: Down syndrome, Fragile X, autism, cystic fibrosis, Marfan syndrome, Prader-Willi syndrome; other conditions such as cerebral palsy, thyroid disease, diabetes, cardiovascular disease; sudden unexplained death, trauma; delayed development of secondary sexual characteristics; sensory deficits, neuromuscular disorders, ethnic background, consanguinity, psychiatric disorders, risky behaviors, trauma.

Questions to explore on cultural concepts of health and illness

1. What would you call this problem?
2. Why do you think your child has developed this problem?
3. What do you think caused the problem?
4. Why do you think the problem started when it did?
5. What do you think is happening inside the body?
6. What are the symptoms that make you know your child has this illness?
7. What are you most worried about with this illness?
8. What problem does this illness cause your child?
9. How do you treat it?
10. Is the treatment helpful?

11. What will happen if this problem is not treated?
12. What do you expect from the treatments?

Please remember that health disparities exist and that culturally sensitive care is imperative to ensure all children have access to the best care available. Refer to the AAP's Policy on Workforce Diversity and Culturally Effective Care of Children (http://pediatrics.aappublications.org/content/pediatrics/132/4/e1105.full.pdf), AAP research on Health Disparities in Young Children (https://www.aap.org/en-us/professional-resources/Research/Pages/Unequal-Treatment-for-Young-Children-Racial-and-Ethnic-Disparities-in-Early-Childhood-Health-and-Healthcare.aspx) and to the ANA's Statement on Diversity (http://www.nursingworld.org/MainMenuCategories/ThePracticeofProfessionalNursing/Improving-Your-Practice/Diversity-Awareness/Mission-Statement.html)

Parenting History:

Other children: ______________________________

Past experience with parenting has been: _____

Type of parenting style used (democratic, autocratic, laissez-faire, etc.) _____

Who are the caregivers?

Discipline techniques used by all caregivers are: _______________

> Note actual or potential interpersonal, social, economic, environmental stresses in family that can affect parenting.

Role expectations of children (boys, girls) are: _____

Safety Issues: This is an opportunity to ask questions about safety, including presence of firearms in the house and any domestic abuse. "Do you feel safe in your home?" should be asked at every visit.

Answers to the aforementioned questions, as well as assessment of the genogram, and family interpersonal relationships can be indicators for potential for abuse. Children can be interviewed without parent/caregiver in an environment that can guarantee safety, protection, and action to help them.

Be sensitive to cultural discipline practices and how they may be perceived.

<u>Sociocultural History</u>: *Many problems in health care can be avoided if provider, patient, and family have the same understanding of words, practices, and expectations. The following information has an impact on the child's physical, emotional, social, cognitive, and developmental health by identifying areas of actual or potential concern.*

Perception of support systems for parent, child, and family are: __________

Perception of type of neighborhood in which family lives, socioeconomic group to which the family identifies, and access and barriers to health care and other services.

Where and with whom does child live? ________________________

Daycare: Yes____ No____ type ____________________, hours spent at daycare per day? Week? ____________________________________

> Note variations in family unit or constellation such as teen parents, cultural issues, adoption, cohabitation, homelessness, parents with special needs, same sex parents, single parent, grandparent(s) or others as primary caregiver(s), or other housemates.

Insurance____________________.

Eligibility: WIC _______________, Food Stamps___________________.

Other forms of public assistance_______________________________________.

<u>Environmental History</u>: Exposure to lead, toxins, cigarettes, radiation; stressful home, abuse or neglect history, lack of stimulation.

Risk of lead exposure from: Home: _______; relative home: _________; daycare: __________; toys/other: __________.

II. Infancy

If possible, arrange a prenatal visit to establish a relationship and discuss specific issues such as genetic history, newborn screening, and care during the first week of life, infant feeding preferences, support systems, living situation, daycare plans, safety, and immunizations.

Prenatal/Perinatal: General areas to be addressed include:

Prenatal history – Lack of/or inadequate prenatal care, exposure to infections such as toxoplasmosis, rubella, cytomegaly virus, herpes simplex, human immunodeficiency virus (HIV); maternal exposure to drugs including over-the-counter (OTC) and complementary medication and/or alcohol, material tobacco use, passive smoke exposure, repeated spontaneous abortions or stillbirths; maternal age >35 years.

Perinatal history – Mode of delivery, medications used, anesthesia, birth trauma, prematurity, fetal distress, trauma or asphyxia at birth, neonatal seizures, jaundice, prolonged labor, low birth weight, meningitis, infections of either the child or mother, poor feeding, and birth defects.

Mother was ____ years old and father was _____ years old at the onset of this pregnancy.

Mother is a Para: _____ Gravida: ______ Living children: ______

There were ______ number of years between this pregnancy and the last.

Mother began antenatal care in the _______ trimester at_______________.

Mother took prenatal vitamins and folic acid as directed. Yes____ No____

Folic acid dose ___

Mother was ______ years old at onset of first menses.

Mother was ______ years old with first pregnancy.

This pregnancy was planned. Yes_____ No______

Mother's primary ethnicity/race is _________; father's______________

HIV testing: Yes_______ No_______ Status: _____ Date: _____________

Mother has ________allergies. Drug: ______; environmental: __________

Father has ________allergies. Drug: ______; environmental: __________

There are _______ pets in the household. Types: _________________

II. Infancy

Mother feels safe. Yes____ No____ Father feels safe. Yes ____ No_____

There are guns/firearms in the house. Yes____ No____ Where are they kept? ____ Are the firearms stored in a child-proof manner? _________

Mother identified the following present during this pregnancy:

Record any pre-existing conditions and maternal illnesses such as gestational diabetes, hypertension, infections including group B strep, urinary tract infections (UTIs), HIV, hepatitis, sexually transmitted infections (STIs), viruses, parasites, maternal syphilis serology urine/blood test abnormalities, blood pressure (BP) problems, bleeding, blood sugar, medications taken including prescription, over-the-counter (OTC), and herbal remedies (past as well), drugs/alcohol exposure, cigarette (active/passive) exposure, exposure to unpasteurized dairy products, undercooked meats, changing cat litter, any other environmental toxin such as lead, mercury, mold; unusual episodes of abdominal pain and contractions, amniotic fluid leak, amniocentesis, ultrasounds, other tests, maternal history for congenital anomaly, genetic disorders, any potential area of concern not mentioned above.

<u>Labor, Delivery, and Postpartum History</u>: *Request copies, if not present on chart, of L&D and postpartum period.*

> Premature or prolonged rupture of membranes, excessively long labor, and/or meconium aspiration increases potential for neonatal and/or maternal infection/sepsis. Reports of fetal distress with anoxia, respiratory, cardiac and neurological disorders noted at birth increase risk of a variety of problems and should be documented.

Mother states labor was ______ hours in length.

When did labor start_________, where was the labor and delivery_________.

When did membranes rupture? _______Color of the amniotic fluid ______.

Labor was induced: Yes _______No_________.

Labor augmented: Yes ________No__________.

Mother required __________________ medication, _________ anesthesia __________________________.

She delivered vaginally ___ or C-section (Include reason for C-section, C-section number) _____.

II. Infancy

Delivery by instrumentation, vacuum or forceps assistance _____

Fetal presentation________________

Episiotomy performed _____or lacerations_________

Record how mother felt about birthing process and what support information was provided.

The following maternal problems occurred after delivery: ____________.

Mother and baby discharged from hospital on day __ post birth.

> Record problems such as fever, infection, bleeding or other abnormal experiences such as mother and child being discharged from hospital on different days

Sociocultural History: *Many problems in health care can be avoided if provider, patient, and family have the same understanding of words, practices, and expectations. The following information has an impact on the child's physical, emotional, social, cognitive, and developmental health by identifying areas of actual or potential concern.*

Perception of support systems for parent, child, and family are: __________.

Perception of type of neighborhood in which family lives, socioeconomic group to which the family identifies, and access and barriers to health care and other services.

Where and with whom does child live? ______________________

Daycare: Yes____ No____ type ___________________, hours spent a daycare per day? Week? _________________________________

Presence of risk of lead exposure from: Home: _______; relative home: ________ daycare: _________

Lead Exposure Risk needs to be assessed for each child−consider risk of any and all residences the child spends time in (home, relatives, daycare). Homes built before 1978 may have lead paint. Please refer to CDC's recommendations http://www.cdc.gov/nceh/lead/

> Note variations in family unit or constellation such as teen parents, cultural issues, adoption, cohabitation, homelessness, parents with special needs, same sex parents, single parent, grandparent(s) or others as primary caregiver(s), or other housemates.

II. Infancy

> Infants are at risk for shaken baby syndrome. Provide counseling and/or reporting according to state rules and regulations.
>
> See National Institute of Neurological Disorders and Stroke/National Institutes of Health (NINDS/NIH) http://www.ninds.nih.gov/disorders/shakenbaby/shakenbaby.htm

Neonate: *Term infants (37 weeks−41 weeks 6 days). Preterm infants (<37 weeks) have increased incidence of hypoglycemia, GE reflux, congenital anomalies, potential for sepsis, hypoxia/anoxia, respiratory distress, bronchopulmonary dysplasia, long-term conditions related to over oxygenation, physiological instability, cerebral bleeds, developmental problems, and cerebral palsy. Post-term infants (≥42 weeks) have increased potential for hypoglycemia, sepsis, dehydration/malnutrition states, polycythemia. Exams should note physiological and developmental status.*

The gestational age at birth of this child was __________ weeks.

Gender: ___________

Birth weight ________ length ______ (adjusted for gestational age as indicated)

Head circumference (HC), term also used, occipital frontal circumference (OFC)

____

Plot on growth chart

This child's Apgar score was ______@ 1 minute ________@ 5 minutes.

Apgar scores @ 1 & 5 minutes <7 have increased potential to be related to a congenital, sepsis, and/or neurological problem. Note any reported fetal distress complications.

Vitamin K prophylaxis given? Yes____ No____

Eye prophylaxis given? Yes____ No____

This child's newborn history includes: _____

> Jaundice, temperature problem, blood group incompatibility, blood sugar problem, infection, respiratory instability, x-rays, blood test, other tests performed, physical exam findings that were suspicious or unusual, i.e., neurologic, cardiac, facies, and meconium stained fluid. Please pay attention to any cultural/ethnic variations.

Infant blood type _________direct Coombs test results________

The PKU and other genetic based testing was drawn __________ and the results were _______________________.

The most accurate PKU is the one drawn after the neonate has been exposed to 48–72 hours of nutritional intake.

Results of NB thyroid screen: __________

A vision screen __________ was performed on ______ or vision status was ascertained by____.

Results of the vision test: _________.

A hearing test was performed on ______ or hearing status was ascertained by____.

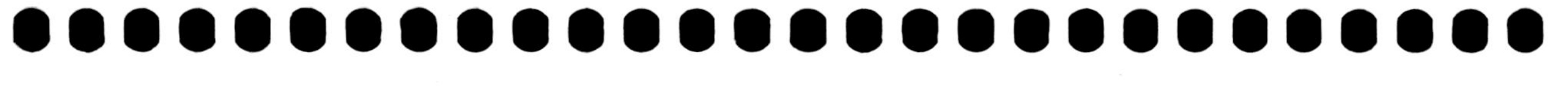

Results of the hearing test: ________.

Neonatal hearing loss can be hereditary, related to maternal virus or medication intake during pregnancy, related to genetic or congenital anomaly universal hearing screens required in most states. Renal anomalies and congenital prolonged QT syndrome can be associated with ear abnormalities and hearing loss.

Newborn transition problems include respiratory distress, cyanosis, hypoglycemia, poor feeding, temperature instability, and jitteriness. Note sleep pattern, elimination pattern with number and type of stools, number of wet diapers in 24 hours.

The ***newborn discharge exam*** identified the presence of the following:

Alertness______

Head shape_____ (size, sutures, fontanels, molding, and trauma)

Normal facies ___

Ocular mobility and red reflex ____ (absence, partial, opacification, ocular mobility)

Intact hard palate ___ (presence of natal teeth, clefts of lip or palate, short frenulum)

Patent ear canals ____ (shape, position in relation to outer canthus, pits or tags)

Patent nasal passage bilaterally ___ (septal deviations)

Pulses in all extremities ___

No evidence of abnormal cardiac findings ___ (rate, rhythm, heart sounds, murmurs)

Hip____ (Ortolani and Barlow maneuvers)

Umbilical cord stump_____

Number of vessels noted in cord at birth ___

Male: Normal genitalia for male _____

Position of urinary meatus at tip of penis, midline? Yes____ No_____

If NO – presence of hypospadias (meatus on ventral surface of glans/penis – 1 in 5000 births)______or presence of epispadias (meatus of dorsal aspect of penis – very rare)___________

Testes descended bilaterally, palpated? Yes____ No_____

Presence of hydrocele: Yes______ bilateral_____ unilateral ______

If present does it increase with position change (communicating) Yes _____ No (stays same size regardless of position or time of day – noncommunicating)______

Circumcised? Yes____ No____

Female: Normal genitalia for female______

Presence of vaginal discharge, labial adhesions? Yes___ No___

II. Infancy

Position of urethral meatus?

Patent anus in male and female?_________ Has infant passed stool since birth?_______ When?__________

Intact spine ____

No foot deformities_______

Normal neonatal reflexes ____

Symmetry of movement_____

Muscle tone______

Presence of birthmarks or skin lesions? Yes_____ No_____ If present, where, size, shape, color? _______

> Presence of a major anomaly, 3 or more minor anomalies, or a combination of both or any recognized pattern of anomalies needs further genetic evaluation.

The infant was breastfed ____bottle fed ____; breast and bottle fed____; type of formula _______ amount_______ frequency______

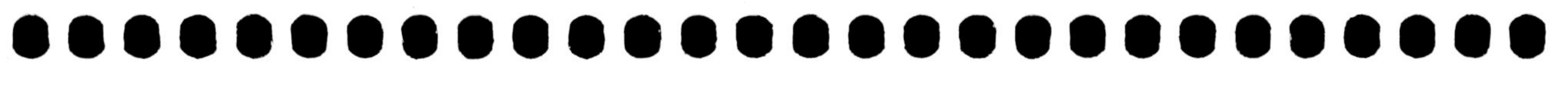

***If breastfed**, record frequency, time on each breast, evidence of feeding difficulties indicative of cardiac problem (as above), difficulty with latch and sucking mechanisms, maternal medications or herbs, evidence of mastitis, altered maternal-child bonding.*

***Breastfeeding** recommended first year of life, for at least 4–6 months if possible. Usually breastfeed 8–12 times per day, eventually as infant matures and sleeps through night 5–6 times per day. Maternal breast milk comes in within 48–72 hours after birth. Prior to milk coming in Mom produces colostrum (high calorie, immunity rich). Advise mother to continue prenatal vitamin while nursing.*

If on vegetarian or vegan diet, also needs additional iron, zinc, and vitamin B_{12}. Advise to avoid alcohol. Give lactation resource. See Quick Reference Chart: Lactation Risk with Medication Category.

If bottle feeding*, record type of formula, quantity, reactions, problems, length of time to feed.* ***Fe fortified formula 1st year****. Evidence of pallor/cyanosis, sweating, respiratory difficulty with feeding or prolonged feeding time (>20 minutes to finish one ounce [29.6 mL]) should be evaluated for cardiac problems. Children in families with history of atopy or in families with potential for or actual lactose intolerance occasionally may need soy based or hypoallergenic formulas.*

General feeding rule: *In the first month of life, an infant needs one hour to digest an ounce (29.6 mL) of formula. Average intake 20 oz/day (0.59 L) neonate; 24−27 oz/day (0.71−0.8 L) 1 month; 26−28 oz/day (0.77−0.83 L) 2 months; 30−32 oz/day (0.89−0.95 L) 4 months.*

Discuss proper preparation, storage and heating of both formula and breast milk. Carefully read directions on formula preparation.

Breastfed and partially breastfed infants should be supplemented with 400 IU a day of vitamin D, beginning in the first few days of life. All non-breastfed infants, as well as older children, who are consuming less than one quart (0.95 L) per day of vitamin D-fortified formula or milk, should receive a vitamin D supplement of 400 IU a day. Adolescents who do not obtain 400 IU of vitamin D per day through foods should receive a supplement containing that amount. Children with increased risk of vitamin D deficiencies, such as those taking certain medications, often need higher vitamin D doses.

Source: AAP Vitamin D Supplementation of Vitamin D https://www.aap.org/en-us/about-the-aap/aap-press-room/Pages/Vitamin-D-Supplementation-for-Infants.aspx; NIH Guidelines for Vitamin D Supplementation https://ods.od.nih.gov/factsheets/VitaminD-HealthProfessional/

Iron storage occurs primarily during 3rd trimester of pregnancy. Preterm infants are at great risk for anemia. Breastfed preterm infants should receive supplemental iron of 2 mg/kg/day and/or through iron rich foods (older infants) from 1 through 12 months. Most full-term infants have sufficient iron stores to maintain health for the first 4–6 months of life, when solid foods are introduced. Infants who receive half or more of their feedings from breast milk should receive an iron supplement of 1 mg/kg/day until they are taking solid iron rich foods. Exclusively formula fed infants should obtain sufficient iron from the formula until iron rich foods are introduced.

All children should be screened for IDA at age 12 months.

Source: "Diagnosis and Prevention of Iron Deficiency and Iron-Deficiency Anemia in Infants and Young Children (0–3 Years of Age)" available at pediatrics.aappublications.org/content/early/2010/10/05/peds.2010-2576.abstract

Use of pacifier: Yes ________ No________

APA finds evidence that pacifier use can help reduce risk of SIDS and should be offered for naps and long-term sleep. Current recommendations state to initiate after breast-feeding (BF) established but newer evidence indicates no interference with BF.

Reference available at: http://www.aappublications.org/content/32/11/1.1

Expected newborn weight loss is 10% of birth weight but should be regained by 2 weeks of age or needs reevaluation.

First follow up newborn visit should occur within 3−5 days after birth and within 48−72 hours after hospital discharge or up to 1 week if C-section delivery and hospital stay 96 hours or longer.

Resources available at: brightfutures.aap.org/continuing_education.html

Evidence of poor feeding, frequent spitting up, coughing while feeding, respiratory problems, color changes such as pallor or dark color, apnea, prolonged crying spells, changes in activity levels, forehead sweating, excessive weight loss or gain. If any of the above is present, consider cardiac, GI problem. Increased hyperbilirubinemia risk in Asian and Native Americans, lower risk with African ancestry

III. Review of Systems and Health Practices

Note who is providing information.

Note interaction between child and parent/guardian.

Obtain parent(s)' name and age(s), # siblings and ages, birth order

Date of birth: ____________________ Gender: __________

Past primary care provider (Name, address if known): ________________________

Date of last health care visit and reason for visit: ______________________________

School/daycare____________, grade/year____________________

If employed, where, # of hours/week, shift? ___________________________________

Has anyone ever told you that you, other family members or your child had a problem with heart, spine, muscles, breathing, or any other body system? If so, what? ____

Any known health problem? ____

Any medications (prescription or over-the-counter)? ___________________________

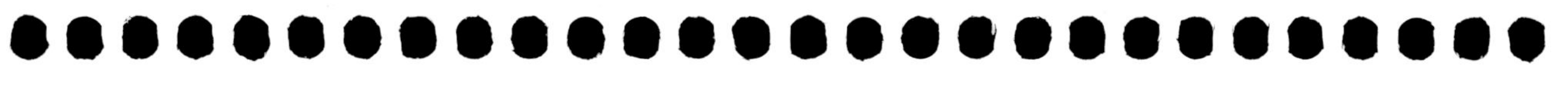

Complementary health practices? (Specifically ask about herbal remedies, vitamin supplements, energy drinks) ________________________________

Allergies (food, drugs, insects, environment): ________________________

Type of reaction: ____________

Epinephrine autoinjector (EpiPen®) use advised? _____ Last use? _____ Location of medication: ________

AAP and AAAI recommend introducing foods associated with allergies (peanut products, tree nuts, cow milk protein, soy, fish, and shellfish) between ages 4–6 months to reduce risk of development of food allergies.

References: Fleischer DM, Spergel JM, Assa'ad AH, Pongracic. J Allergy Clin Immunol: In Practice 2013;1:29-36.; https://www.aaaai.org/Aaaai/media/MediaLibrary/PDF%20Documents/Libraries/Preventing-Allergies-15.pdf

New interim recommendations based on recent evidence indicating that decreased peanut allergies with early introduction (between 4–6 months of age) of peanut products to high risk infants. Definitive EBP guidelines due for release in 2017. Interim guidelines found at http://www.jacionline.org/article/ S0091-6749%2815%2900785-X/full

No nuts or popcorn <4 years of age due to safety or choking risk.

Carefully evaluate drug responses, which may only be medication sensitivity, a drug-illness interaction effect, and not an allergic reaction.

Immunizations: *Current immunization schedules are available yearly through the Advisory Committee on Immunization Practices (ACIP) Centers for Disease Prevention and Control (www.cdc.gov/vaccines) and American Academy of Pediatrics (www.aap.org). Clinician must be well-informed about the recommended regular and catch-up immunization schedule as well as what immunizations are required before entry into school, what immunizations are given in the presence of immunocompromise, what immunizations are recommended for high risk population, immigrants, and children of international adoption. See Quick Reference Chart: Immunization (IZ) Reaction.*

Focused Visit: Note reason for current visit.

Acute Presenting Problem:

Chief complaint: The child/adolescent and/or historian says the reason for the visit is: _____

History of present illness (HPI):

Symptom analysis– *characteristics of a symptom*

O – Onset; gradual or sudden? ____________

L – Location of symptom; where did it start, where did it progress to, where does it radiate? ___________________

D – Duration; How long has the symptom been present? Is it worsening, improving, unchanged? Symptoms constant, recurrent, intermittent? ________

C – Characteristic/quality of symptom; aching, throbbing, stabbing, burning? _____________

A – Aggravating factors– what makes it worse? _____________

R – Relieving– what makes it better? What treatment has been tried and how has it worked? ____________

T – Timing; any worsening or improvement related to time of day or night? ____________

S – Associated symptoms: Fever, nausea, vomiting, rash, headache, weakness, others, impact of ADLs, perception of illness? _______________

Chronic Health Problem:

Onset and chronology of problem (Date of initial diagnosis with initial symptoms, how and where diagnosed, initial treatment and response, current treatment and response if different from initial, sequelae, specialist involved and frequency of visits, restrictions, special needs)

Such data gives essential information about longevity of problem, change in symptomatology, steady state of the problem, associated problems, multiagency involvement, and potential impact on family dynamics, available support and resources, primary care needs of the child/adolescent.

Past Health History:

Request records to assist with primary care of child/adolescent.

Hospitalizations: Date, facility, provider, problem, outcome/sequelae

Surgeries: Date, facility, provider, procedure, complications, outcome/sequelae

Fractures: Age, type, bone involved, cause, provider, complications, outcome/sequelae

Significant injuries/illnesses: Date, diagnosis, intervention, complications, outcome/sequelae

Therapies for chronic condition: Medications both prescription and OTC, nutritional needs, rehabilitation, equipment, special education, activity restrictions, complementary modalities

Immunizations: Dates, reactions

Allergies: Dates, reactions

Blood transfusions: Dates, reason for transfusion, reactions

Traumas: Dates, description

Significant viral illnesses have increased potential for sequelae i.e., Guillain-Barré syndrome, connective tissue disorders, diabetes mellitus, idiopathic thrombocytopenia (ITP), nephrosis, hepatitis, and immunocompromised states. Significant antibiotic reactions include erythema multiforme, Stevens-Johnson syndrome, erythema nodosum, *C. difficile*-associated diarrhea, colitis.

History of significant injuries, concussions, and overuse syndromes predisposes the patient to orthopedic problems at a later date.

History of concussions predispose to neurological symptoms and possible serious sequelae, especially if reinjured within short time interval

Source: Rice, S.G. and the Council on Sports Medicine and Fitness (2008). Medical conditions affecting sports participation: *Pediatrics, 121 (4),* 841–848. Policy reaffirmed 2010 by AAP. Available at: https://pediatrics.aappublications.org/content/pediatrics/121/4/841.full.pdf

Resources for athletes, parents and providers available at: http://www.stopsportsinjuries.org

M. Tombasco, W. Wright, *Expert Exam: Conducting a Pre-sports Physical Examination*, Fitzgerald Health Education Associates, North Andover, MA. Available at fhea.com

History of childhood illnesses/infections such as, varicella, mononucleosis, rheumatoid disease, or such conditions as mumps, rubella, measles, pertussis, tuberculosis (TB) exposure, BCG vaccine. Children who are inadequately immunized are at risk to acquiring and transmitting these diseases.

Developmental History: Note any illness, medication history of child/adolescent, failure to thrive, failure to achieve milestones, decreased interests in surroundings, feeding problems, food or formula intolerance, speech and language delay, abnormal behavior; school performance: Distractibility, short attention span, and difficulty following directions.

Habits: Exercise, nutrition, vitamin supplements, sports drinks, sleep, hygiene, structured vs. unstructured activities, caffeine (coffee, soda, energy drinks) intake, alcohol/drug experiences, tobacco, marijuana (personal use or exposure to use by others).

AAP Clinical Report on energy and sports drinks recommends the following: Sports drinks should be avoided for all children and adolescents in general due to high caloric content and only used in certain limited situations.

Energy drinks are not recommended and should be avoided for all children and adolescents due to the potentially dangerous stimulant side effects.

Resource available at: pediatrics.aappublications.org/content/early/2011/05/25/peds.2011-0965

Body image, self-esteem, family dynamics, family history for eating disorders are important variables that can impact this child/adolescent's health maintenance practices.

Pressure for athletics, musical, school excellence increases potential for eating disorders, anabolic steroid use/abuse, and other substance use/abuse.

Sleep problems can be developmental but if not dealt with appropriately may lead to long-term insomnia and physiological sequelae.

Safety:

Ask about the following issues:

1. Seatbelts, car seats, booster seats (type, appropriateness of seat restraint for age/size of child). See Quick Reference Chart: *Car Safety Seat Use*. See www.nhtsa.gov (http://www-odi.nhtsa.dot.gov/owners/SearchSafetyIssues?prodType=C) for specific car seat safety and *Car Seats: Information for Families* available at www.healthychildren.org/English/safety-prevention/on-the-go/pages/Car-Safety-Seats-Information-for-Families.aspx or www.seatcheck.org; may also call **866/SEATCHECK** (866-732-8243); http://safeseats4kids.aaa.com/car-seat-guide/
2. Other motor vehicle safety– Motorcycle, dirt bike, ATV, snowmobile, personal watercraft (i.e., Jet Ski®), etc.
3. Presence of guns in house (gun and ammunition storage safety, locked, use of guns)

4. Bicycle helmets, roller-blade, skateboarding, snowboarding pads/helmets, mouth guards; available at www.healthychildren.org/English/safety-prevention/at-play/pages/How-To-Get-Your-Child-To-Wear-a-Bicycle-Helmet.aspx
5. Presence of smoke detectors, carbon monoxide detectors, radon detectors, sprinklers
6. Presence of family fire escape plan; available at www.usfa.fema.
7. Water heater temperature set at $\leq$120°F (49°C); bath water between 90°−100°F (32°−38°C)
8. Lead paint and dust lead levels evaluated in homes built before 1978 (See www.epa.gov for additional information; lead paint remediation: https://www.epa.gov/lead/steps-lead-safe-renovation-repair-and-painting-october-2011). Air purifiers, humidifiers, wood-burning stoves, appliances to heat house
9. Child-proofed house as age-appropriate

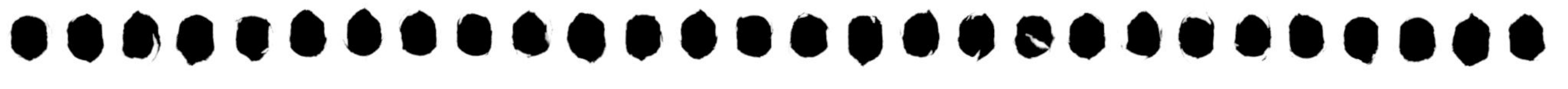

10. Occupational exposures that can bring substances home (fertilizer, asbestos, paint, chemicals, smoke, additional information at www.epa.gov)
11. Stranger protection (family codes, emergency procedures, telephone/online safety)
12. Poison control center phone number: 1-800-222-1222
13. Food safety, no nuts or popcorn <4 years old

References: Fleischer DM, Spergel JM, Assa'ad AH, Pongracic. ***J Allergy Clin Immunol: In Practice*** **2013;1:29-36.; https://www.aaaai.org/Aaaai/media/MediaLibrary/PDF%20Documents/Libraries/Preventing-Allergies-15.pdf**

14. Personal safety from physical, emotional, verbal, sexual abuse
15. Bully, victim, playground/school safety
16. Potential risks at home, yard, and neighborhood

Find AAP recommendations for safety at www.healthychildren.org/English/safety-prevention/Pages/default.aspx

General Health Screening: Based on U.S. Preventive Services Task Force (USPSTF) *The Guide to Clinical Preventive Services: Report of the United States Preventive Services Task Force* available at: http://www.ahrq.gov/professionals/clinicians-providers/guidelines-recommendations/guide/index.html and Recommendations for Preventive Pediatric Health Care found in *Bright Futures Guidelines for Health Supervision of Infants, Children and Adolescents*: American Academy of Pediatrics; available at: brightfutures.aap.org

Assessment of growth and development occurs at two levels, combining formal screening with informal observations, repeated measures at different ages and use of multiple sources of information particularly parental report. Generally, there are 6 domains of development to explore:

Gross motor, fine motor, language, psychosocial, cognitive, and physical.

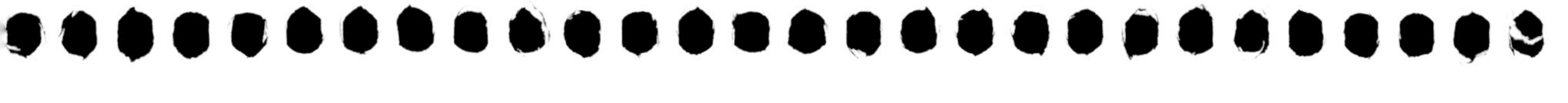

Developmental surveillance includes evaluation of physical growth of the child/adolescent, recognition of "red flags" which indicate possible abnormal development or at risk development, and acceptance of normal developmental variations.

Sources: www.cdc.gov/ncbddd/childdevelopment/index.html; Bright Futures Guidelines for Health Supervision of *Infants, Children and Adolescents*: American Academy of Pediatrics; available at: brightfutures.aap.org

See Quick Reference Charts: Early Childhood Growth, Anticipated Early Childhood Developmental Milestones, Language Milestones.

Growth:

Weight

Length until age 2 years then standing height after 3 years

HC or OFC until age 3 years

Chest circumference until 1 year

Plot on growth charts: Abnormal growth is considered <5% for height and weight; macrocephaly >90% head circumference (OFC), microcephaly, <5%. Parental growth parameters (especially head circumference) and dysmorphic features should also be assessed. www.cdc.gov/growthcharts

Skinfold Thickness:

BMI >2 years

Body Mass Index (BMI) is a number calculated from a child's weight and height. BMI is a reliable indicator of body fatness for most children and teens. For children and teens, BMI is age- and sex-specific and is often referred to as BMI-for-age www.cdc.gov/healthyweight/assessing/bmi/

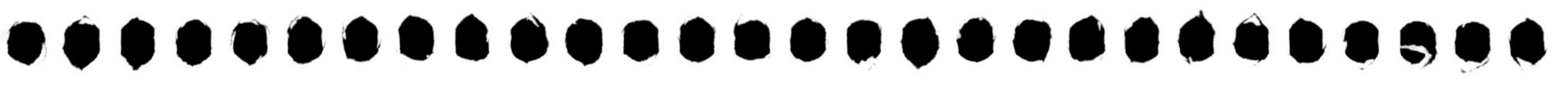

Blood Pressure Screen:

Children age ≥3 years should be checked at every health care visit, whether well or unwell. The preferred BP measurement is auscultation.

Children less than 3 years of age should have BP checked if there is a history of prematurity, very low birth weight, a NICU stay, congenital heart disease, recurrent urinary tract infections, renal disease, organ transplant, treatment with drugs that increase BP, systemic illness with hypertension, and increased intracranial pressure.

Average systolic and diastolic readings on repeated measurements below 90% for age, gender, and height. All children whose blood pressures are greater than 95th percentile need further evaluation. Additional information: A Pocket Guide to BP Measurement in Children (https://www.nhlbi.nih.gov/files/docs/bp_child_pocket.pdf) and for at risk children; *Ambulatory Blood Pressure Monitoring in Children and Adolescents: Recommendations for Standard Assessment*, available at http://hyper.ahajournals.org/content/63/5/1116

<u>Vision Screen</u>:

Routine screening for amblyopia, strabismus and refractive error, birth to 5 years

Red reflex– Neonates/infants

15 months visit– Cover eye test-conjugate ocular mobility

3-, 4-, 5-, 6-year visit– Visual acuity screen and ophthalmoscopic exam of optic nerve and retina vessels then every 2 years through age 10 years, then once 11–14 years, 15–17 years, and 18–21 years.

AAP policy on vision and ophthalmological screening by pediatric primary care providers available at: pediatrics.aappublications.org/content/111/4/902

<u>Hearing Screen</u>:

Newborn screening recommended for all infants, mandated most states.

4-, 5-, 6-year visits audiometry then every 2 years through 10 years

Early Hearing Detection and Intervention Program **available at: https://www.aap.org/en-us/advocacy-and-policy/aap-health-initiatives/PEHDIC/pages/early-hearing-detection-and-intervention.aspx**

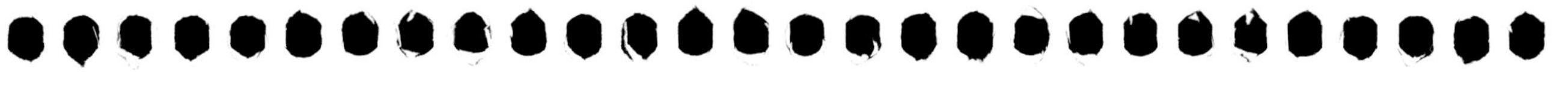

Dental Screen:

Oral health risk assessment 6 months, 9 months

12 months formal dental care or beginning with presence of first tooth, then every 6 months. Healthy Children oral health guidelines available at: https://www.healthychildren.org/English/healthy-living/oral-health/Pages/Brushing-Up-on-Oral-Health-Never-Too-Early-to-Start.aspx and Bright Futures: Oral Health Resource: https://brightfutures.aap.org/Bright%20Futures%20Documents/8-Promoting_Oral_Health.pdf

First tooth ___ age ______, # primary teeth _____, # permanent teeth____, # molars_______

Breastfed or bottle fed____________

After 1 year water only in bottle, limit juice and give in cup only

Fluoride: Check with local public health department on fluoridated water supply and if possible with dentist regarding caries risk. ADA policy states that only those children older than 6 months and no older than 16 years who are at risk for dental caries.

ADA Resource available at http://www.ada.org/en/public-programs/advocating-for-the-public/fluoride-and-fluoridation

Recommendations for fluoride supplementation available at: www.cdc.gov/mmwr/preview/mmwrhtml/rr5014a1.htm#tab1

7 years orthodontia referral if indicated.

Dentist is _________; visit schedule is _____, dental problems________.

Guidelines for infant oral health and assessment available at: http://www.aapd.org/media/policies_guidelines/g_infantoralhealthcare.pdf

CDC resource for promoting oral health and preventing oral diseases available at: http://www.cdc.gov/OralHealth/index.htm

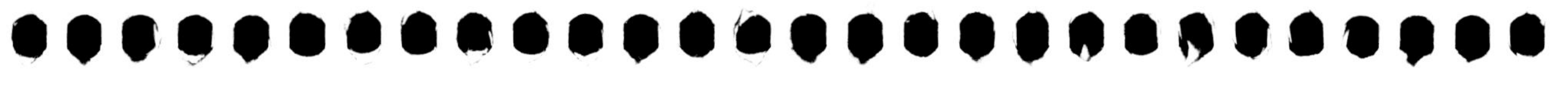

Cholesterol Screen:

Universal screening with fasting lipid profile (FLP) or nonfasting lipid profile (NFLP) ***all*** *children once between ages 9−11 years and once between 18−21 years, regardless of personal or family history.*

FLP or NFLP between 2−21 years, all children with positive family history of dyslipidemia or premature cardiovascular disease, all children with unknown history (i.e., adoption, immigrant) or other risk factors (i.e., BMI>85%, HTN, smoking, dyslipidemia, or diabetes)

NHLBP-NIH Guidelines for CV Screening in Children and Adolescents available at:

http://www.nhlbi.nih.gov/health-pro/guidelines/current/cardiovascular-health-pediatric-guidelines/summary

Hct/Hgb Screen:

First level age 1 year or more often if child at risk. Date & result: _____

Urine Screen:

Not recommended unless at risk; i.e., fever of unknown origin (FUO), symptoms, history renal problems

Tuberculosis (Tb) Screen: Historical review for at risk only.

Is the child/adolescent infected with HIV?

Is the child/adolescent incarcerated?

Has a family member/contact had Tb or a positive Tb skin test?

Was the child/adolescent born in or traveled to a high-risk country >1 week?

Screening, diagnosing, and treatment guidelines available at: www.cdc.gov/tb/publications/LTBI/default.htm

Date & results if PPD given: _____

Date & results of chest x-ray if indicated: ________

Date of BCG if received: _________

Lead Screen:

Environmental screen each visit. Screen blood lead levels (BLL) at 12 months and 24 months. Check additional state requirements. *If child is developmentally delayed, likely will require continued screening depending on behavioral risk.*

Date & results if lead level drawn: 1 year ________ 2 year__________

Screen for lead risk: Developmental delay_____ Age of residences/daycare setting (<1978)_______

> More frequently if BLL elevated and other risk factor identified by Environmental Protection Agency (EPA) questionnaire available at http://www2.epa.gov/lead; resource for providers and parents at https://blogs.cdc.gov/yourhealthyourenvironment/2015/10/26/lead-free-kids-national-lead-poisoning-prevention-week-2015/
>
> CDC National Center for Environmental Health Lead program. State and local programs available at www.cdc.gov/HealthyHomes/programs.html
>
> See Quick Reference Chart: *Managing Elevated Blood Lead Levels Among Young Children.*

Other Environmental Screen: As indicated per risk

STI, Cervical Cancer Screening:

Have you had sex (describe activity)? Yes _______ No ______

Consensual? ____________

Sexual orientation? __________

Type of activity; vaginal ______ anal _____ oral ________

Number of intimate partners_________

Age of partners _______

Condom use? Yes____ No____

Other birth control use? ________

Aware of availability and efficacy of emergency contraception? ________

Are you interested in having a child? ________If so, when? _________

Cervical cancer screening (Pap test) should begin at age 21 regardless of previous sexual history. (Available at: http://www.cancer.org/cancer/cervicalcancer/moreinformation/cervicalcancerpreventionandearlydetection/cervical-cancer-prevention-and-early-detection-cervical-cancer-screening-guidelines)

Pap test if indicated. Date & result: _____

Screening for STIs done? For what type STIs? ________Date: _________ Result: __________

If positive what treatment was given? ________Treatment completed? Yes_____ No____ Partner treated? Yes_____ No____

Screening for HIV: ________ Date: ______ Result: ____

CDC recommends yearly routine screening of sexually active females ≤25 years for *C. trachomatis* and *N. gonorrhoeae.* Males seen at teen/STD clinics, correctional facilities should be screened also. More extensive screening recommended for pregnant teens and young men who have sex with men (YMSM). CDC also recommends universal voluntary HIV screening for all sexually active and high-risk people, beginning at age 13 years.

Resource available at: www.cdc.gov/mmwr/preview/mmwrhtml/rr5912a1.htm

See CDC's website for mobile apps– STD treatment app is just one of many tools that are updated regularly: http://www.cdc.gov/mobile/mobileapp.html#S

Consider testing for syphilis, hepatitis B (HBV) and C (HCV), HIV, and other STIs as indicated. Update HPV, HBV vaccines as needed.

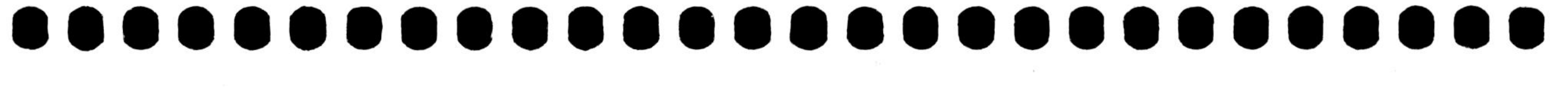

Mental Health Assessment:

Enhancing Pediatric Mental Health Care: Algorithms for Primary Care

Jane Meschan Foy and for the American Academy of Pediatrics Task Force on Mental Health Pediatrics 2010;125;S109-S125

The online version of this article, along with updated information and services, is available at: pediatrics.aappublications.org/content/125/Supplement_3/S109.full

Bright Futures Mental Health Tool Kit, available at: www.brightfutures.org/mentalhealth/pdf/tools.html#professionals

USPSTF Guidelines for Clinical Preventive Practice available at http://www.ahrq.gov/health-care-information/topics/topic-mental-health-childadolescent.html

NAPNAP Mental Health Resources available at: https://www.napnap.org/mental-health-facts

Maternal Depression: Screen at newborn and 6 wk visit. Edinburgh Postnatal Depression Scale (EPDS) available at: www.fresno.ucsf.edu/pediatrics/downloads/edinburghscale.pdf

Child/Adolescent Depression: A validated tool, the Patient Health Questionnaire (PHQ) consists of 9 questions (PHQ-9) that can screen for depression. The first two questions of the Patient Health Questionnaire (Questions 1 & 2) are referred to as the PHQ-2, can be used without the remaining 7 questions to assess depressed mood and anhedonia. A positive response to both of these questions is highly correlated to depression. Available at: www.apa.org/pi/about/publications/caregivers/practice-settings/assessment/tools/patient-health.aspx

PHQ-2: Over the past 2 weeks have you been bothered by:

1. Little interest or pleasure in doing things
2. Feeling down, depressed, or hopeless

PHQ-9

3. Trouble falling or staying asleep, or sleeping too much
4. Feeling tired or having little energy
5. Poor appetite or overeating

6. Feeling bad about yourself or that you are a failure or have let yourself or your family down
7. Trouble concentrating on things, such as reading the newspaper or watching TV
8. Moving or speaking so slowly that other people could have noticed? Or the opposite – being so fidgety or restless that you have been moving around a lot more than usual
9. Thoughts that you would be better off dead or hurting yourself in some way

<u>Infant/Toddler Screen</u>: Patterns of attachment; shaken baby syndrome; Autism Spectrum Screen in development surveillance 15 mo visit

Specific tool– Pediatric Symptom Checklist (PSC) 18 mos. and 24 mos.; child maltreatment, discipline and behavioral issues, available at: https://brightfutures.org/development/early/overview_screening.html

Autism Spectrum Disorder Screen:

MCHAT tool available at: http://www2.gsu.edu/~psydlr/M-CHAT/Official_M-CHAT_Website_files/M-CHAT-R_F.pdf

See Quick Reference Chart: ***Developmental "Red Flags" In the Young Child***

Early Childhood/School-age: Connectedness, learning disorders, bullying/victim, conduct disorders, depression, anxiety, bipolar disorders, ADHD

Adolescent Substance Abuse Screen: All adolescents should be screened for tobacco, alcohol, and other drug use and an anti-tobacco message should be counseled at each visit.

Tobacco Screening:

Screen for Environmental Tobacco Smoke (ETS) exposure at 1 month, 2 month, and 7–21 year visits, and tobacco use at 11–21 year visits.

Alcohol/Drug Screen:

CRAFFT Questions* *A Brief Screening Test for Adolescent Substance Abuse*

- **C** = Have you ever ridden in a CAR driven by someone (including yourself) who was "high" or had been using alcohol or drugs?
- **R** = Do you ever use alcohol or drugs to RELAX, feel better about self or to fit in?
- **A** = Do you ever use alcohol/drugs while you are by yourself, ALONE?
- **F** = Do you FORGET things you did while using alcohol or drugs?
- **F** = Do your family or FRIENDS ever tell you that you should cut down on your drinking or drug use?
- **T** = Have you gotten into TROUBLE while you were using alcohol or drugs?

*2 or more yes answers suggests a significant problem

Source: http://www.ceasar-boston.org/CRAFFT/

HEADSS Assessment of:

Home environment and family relations

Educational environment, teachers, friends

Activities (social, sports, extracurricular, dating)

Depression (eating, sleeping, friends, sadness)

Sex (maturation, sexual activity, safe sex, birth control, etc.)

Suicide (thoughts, ideation, plan, acts)

Policy and guidelines for prevention and identification of substance abuse, tobacco use, and high risk behaviors using history, observation, and surveillance available through *A Bright Futures Handbook.* Available at: https://brightfutures.aap.org/materials-and-tools/PerfPrevServ/Pages/default.aspx

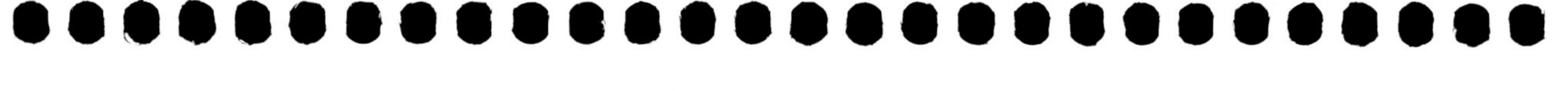

Self-concept, Body Image, Self-esteem:

Inability to identify strengths in the areas may indicate depression, parent/caregiver dysfunction, abuse, or poor resilience potential.

School performance: Grades, days missed, activities, friends, and sports.

Stress:

Personality type, reaction to stress, levels of stress, types of stress, coping strategies; provide mentoring for overcoming stress/adversities, self-comforting abilities, self-amusement activities

How do you cope with stress?

How are you helping your child/adolescent become a good decision maker and cope with stress?

Support Systems:

Friends, family, teachers, coaches, groups, teams, opportunities for socialization, lack of support increases risk for poor resilience, depression, suicide

Cultural/Socioeconomic:

Finances

Source of income, inadequate income, need for financial assistance, number of dependents, living accommodations and adequacy to meet family needs, perception of social class to which family belongs. Qualify for WIC/food stamps, other public assistance?

Cultural Practices

Illness/wellness beliefs and practices, use of complementary modalities and healers, religious influences, ethnic/racial preferences, communication (language, need for interpreter), discipline techniques, infant/child sleeping arrangements, role expectations of family members, perception of healthcare system and healthcare provider.

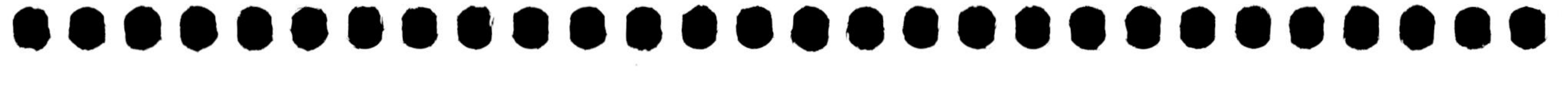

General History:

History of frequent, unexplained fevers: Consider HIV, cancers, Hodgkin disease or other lymphoma, leukemia.

History of malaise, weakness, fatigue: Symptoms possibly representative of mononucleosis, fibromyalgia, hypothyroidism, infection, sleep deprivation, depression, mental health issues, eating disorders, cancer.

Weight loss or gain: Can be indicative of hypo/hyperthyroidism, diabetes, HIV, cancer, inflammatory bowel disease, nephrosis/nephritis, heart failure, depression.

Skin:

Color Changes

Can indicate perfusion problems, cardiac problems, Raynaud's syndrome, jaundice.

Dryness

Can be nutritional deficits, atopic dermatitis response, hypothyroidism.

Lesions and Masses

May be injuries, tumors, cysts, secondary skin lesions, moles, precancerous lesions.

Rashes

Possibly related to dermatitis, drug effect, illness reaction, bleeding phenomenon, or may be fungal, candida, warts that may or may not be early signs of infectious disease. See Quick Reference Chart: *Acute, Febrile, Rash-producing Illness*.

Itchiness

Possibly related to dermatitis reaction or scabies. Examine for drug/virus/illness.

<u>Hair</u>:

Hair color is_____, evenly distributed, appropriate to chronological age.

Loss of Hair

Possibly related to malnutrition, alopecia from trauma, stress, self-injury, parasitic infestation, hypothyroidism, fungal infection.

Hair Shaft Damage

From use of dyes, perms, straighteners, ponytails/pigtails too tight (traction alopecia), vitamin deficiency, medications, parasitic infestation, fungal infection.

<u>Nails</u>:

Nails are appropriate in color and texture.

Thickened yellow nails from fungal infection (onychomycosis), spoon nails from iron deficiency, clubbing from chronic oxygen deficiency, pitting due to psoriasis, damage from artificial nails, nail biting, could be at risk for parasitic infestation, anxiety disorders.

Head and Face:

Headaches

Migraines can begin in preschool and school-age years. Can also indicate visual problem, hypoglycemia reactions, increased intracranial pressure and/or associated with anxiety, school problems, or other social problems.

Facial Pain

Usually indicates dental problem, sinusitis, neurological problem, Lyme disease, temporomandibular joint (TMJ) disorder, or trauma.

Eyes:

Eyes, lids, and conjunctiva appear normal. Funduscopic exam is normal.

> Excessive eye rubbing can indicate itchiness, allergies, and visual problems.

Redness, Discharge, Excessive Tearing

Note if unilateral, color, frequency, amount.

> Possibly related to conjunctivitis, stress hemorrhage, corneal abrasion, iritis, dacryocystitis, or lacrimal stenosis.

Swelling of Lids

> Possibly related to edema, hordeolum, or chalazion. Associated with renal problems.

Cloudiness or Whiteness of Cornea

> Possibly related to cataract, congenital glaucoma, or retinoblastoma.

Ears:

Pain

Possibly related to otitis externa, otitis media, eustachian tube congestion, presence of foreign body, abrasion of canal from use of object to clean ears.

Earwax

Cerumen is a natural product that should not be routinely removed unless impacted. The ears should be cleaned only when enough earwax accumulates to cause symptoms or interferes/prevents a needed assessment of the ear.

Impacted cerumen may cause one or more of the following symptoms: Earache, fullness in the ear, or a sensation the ear is plugged, partial hearing loss, which may be progressive, tinnitus, ringing, or noises in the ear, itching, odor, or discharge, coughing; water may get trapped behind and around impaction causing irritation/inflammation of canal and TM

Source: The American Academy of Otolaryngology – Head and Neck Surgery Foundation (AAO-HNSF) Clinical Practice Guideline: Cerumen Impaction, available at http://oto.sagepub.com/content/139/3_suppl_1/S1.full.pdf+html

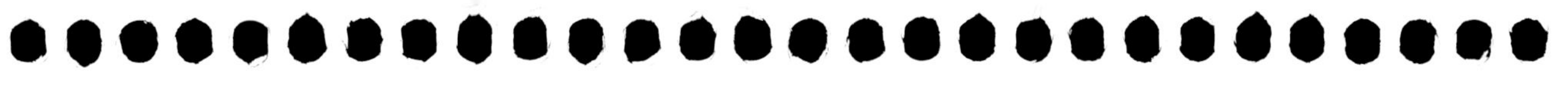

Discharge

Possibly related to perforated tympanic membrane, otitis externa, or foreign body.

Hearing Problems

Possibly related to ceruminosis, cystic formation in canal, foreign body, chronic otitis media with effusion, conductive or sensory hearing loss, or cholesteatoma.

Nose/Sinuses:

External Lesions of Nose

Possibly related to impetigo or herpes simplex, or in older children/adolescents it may be cancerous skin lesion or infection from piercing

Nasal Discharge

One-sided usually purulent indicative of foreign body in nasal passage. Clear/white rhinorrhea indicative of viral or allergic rhinitis. Purulent (yellow or green) can be indicative of bacterial infective process in airway system (throat, sinuses, ears).

Nasal Pain

Possibly related to sinusitis, dryness, or secondary to cocaine or other substance sniffing.

Itchiness, Sneezing, and "Salute" Sign

Usually related to allergies (often sneezing bouts first sign of asthma with or without wheezing).

Nosebleeds

Possibly related to nasal congestion, irritation usually from picking, evident when using inhaled drugs, first sign of a bleeding or coagulation problem in patient or foreign body.

Mouth/Lips/Throat:

Pain on Lips, in Mouth, Gums, Tongue, Throat

Possibly related to nutrition issues or mouth breathing due to congestion or adenoids. May indicate dental abscess, strep throat, viral illness, herpes, Coxsackie virus, aphthous ulcer.

Lesions

Possibly related to viral infection (Coxsackie, herpetic), or cancerous lesions (especially in adolescents who chew tobacco).

Bleeding and Edema of Gums

Possibly related to gingivostomatitis, vitamin B_{12} deficiency, periodontal disease, bleeding disorder, nutritional issues, anemia, or infection.

Tooth Pain

Possibly indicative of teething, dental caries, malocclusion, malalignment, TMJ disease, or trauma.

Halitosis

Possibly related to an infectious process (bacterial, viral, fungal) poor dental hygiene, foreign body in nose or sinusitis.

Neck/Lymph Nodes:

Stiffness or Pain

Possibly related to torticollis, cervical strain, trauma, stress, meningitis, lymphadenopathy, or lymphadenitis.

Masses, Swelling, and Tenderness

Mass can indicate enlarged lymph nodes, thyroid nodule, goiter, Hodgkin disease or other lymphoma (especially if present in clavicular area), mumps, or mononucleosis.

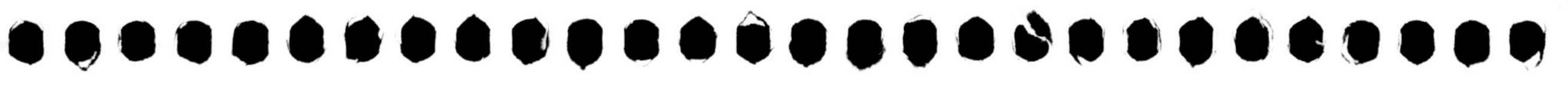

Breasts:

Swelling

Possibly related to newborn hormonal response, adolescent gynecomastia in males, obesity-related gynecomastia, breast budding in pubescent females, pregnancy, steroid or drug use.

Tenderness

Possibly related to peri-menses hormonal effect, mastitis, cyst, injury, breast mass (benign or malignant), pregnancy, fibrocystic breast disease. Evidence largely anecdotal for high caffeine intake contributing to breast pain.

Discharge

In female teen, consider pregnancy, mastitis, malignancy. Possibly related to hormonal response in newborns. Consider both illegal and prescription drug use including marijuana, second generation antipsychotic use.

<u>Breast Cancer Screening</u>:

Breast self-examination (BSE)

Should be encouraged to assist young girls to learn more about general health of breasts. However not indicated for cancer screening.

Beginning in their early 20s, women should be told about the benefits and limitations of BSE. The importance of prompt reporting of any new breast symptoms to a health professional should be emphasized. Women who choose to do BSE should receive instruction and have their technique reviewed on the occasion of a periodic health examination. It is acceptable for women to choose not to do BSE or to do BSE irregularly.

Clinical breast examination (CBE)

The ACS does not recommend clinical breast examination for breast cancer screening among average-risk women at any age.

Available at: http://jama.jamanetwork.com/article.aspx?articleid=2463262

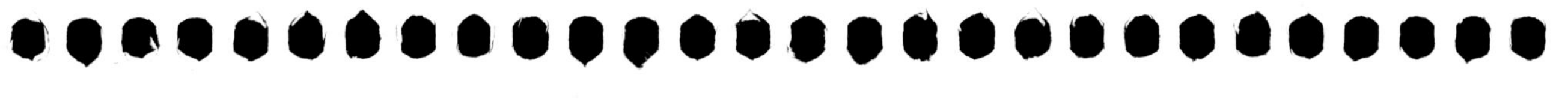

Respiratory:

Cough

Identifying frequency, sputum production, presence of fever, time of cough.

Possibly related to post-nasal drip vs. viral vs. bacterial vs. pertussis infections. Clear or white sputum production usually presents with viral infections; yellow or green sputum suggests bacterial infection. Bloody sputum is usually indicative of epistaxis or tuberculosis. May be sign of gastroesophageal reflux disease (GERD).

Wheezing

Evident as a reactive airway process in most pediatric diseases such as bronchiolitis, bronchitis, pneumonia, and asthma. May also be referred sounds from congested nasal breathing. Medications such as erythromycin, clarithromycin, and ciprofloxacin can alter the metabolism of theophylline which can increase the bronchodilator effect of bronchodilators used in the management of asthma need careful consideration. See Quick Reference Chart: *Differential Diagnosis of Wheeze in Children*.

Respiratory Distress or Presence of Stridor

Evident in significant airway obstructive processes (laryngeal, tracheal, bronchial areas).

In either condition above remember to consider the presence of a foreign body.

Consider apnea, hypertrophic tonsils and/or adenoids.

See Quick Reference Chart: *Differential Diagnosis of Stridor in Children.*

Cardiac:

Chest Pain

Possibly related to pneumonia, asthma, spontaneous pneumothorax (adolescent male most frequently), pulmonary emboli, carditis, or palpitations (related to excessive caffeine intake, anxiety, hyperthyroidism, supraventricular tachycardia (SVT), gastritis, gastroesophageal reflux, prolonged QT syndrome, or musculoskeletal problem (costochondritis).

Murmurs

Majority are physiological or innocent in childhood. However, the presence of some murmurs warrant referral to a cardiac specialist for assessment, especially if audible in diastole, after exercise, or when there is no change in murmur with change in position from supine to stand or squat to stand maneuver or with report of activity intolerance or other low cardiac output symptoms. Ascertain need for antimicrobial prophylaxis, required in the presence of some but not all cardiac murmurs.

ACC/AHA Guideline Update on Valvular Heart Disease: Focused Update on Infective Endocarditis. Available at: http://content.onlinejacc.org/article.aspx?articleid=1838843

Cyanotic and acyanotic congenital heart defects may be present.

Syncope

Possibly indicates cardiac arrhythmias, hypotensive states, heart block, cardiac outflow blockage, hypertrophic cardiomyopathy, high grade aortic stenosis, prolonged QT syndrome, hypoglycemia, seizure, or hyperventilation.

Other Symptoms

Prolonged feeding with sweating or poor suck in infant can indicate congenital heart disease and congestive heart failure. Unequal pulses in extremities may indicate coarctation of the aorta. Tachycardia is often noted in hyperthyroidism, VT, SVT, with select drug adverse effect such as theophylline or aspirin overdose, fever response, anemia, or be present in tachypnea and respiratory distress.

ADHD

See guidelines – Vitter, V. et al. AHA Guidelines: Cardiovascular Monitoring of Children and Adolescents with Heart Disease Receiving Medications for Attention Deficit/Hyperactivity Disorder available at http://circ.ahajournals.org/content/117/18/2407.extract

Hematological:

Bruising & Prolonged Bleeding

Post viral idiopathic thrombocytopenia purpura (ITP), congenital or acquired bleeding disorder, anemia, cancer, ASA or NSAID overuse/overdose, Henoch-Schönlein purpura, or trauma.

Anemia

Most likely anemia in childhood is iron deficiency. Additional anemias to consider include: Thalassemia, G6PD, sickle-cell, folate deficiency, and lead poisoning.

Tattoos, Piercings, Brandings

Continued risk for HIV, hepatitis B & C

Gastrointestinal:

Appetite & Weight

Loss of appetite can be normal during developmental slow periods, can also indicate anemia, illness, cancer, psychological anorexia, hypothyroidism, heat reaction, pharyngitis, dental disease.

Inappropriately increased appetite can indicate learned behavior, physical response to exercise, hyperthyroidism, depression, or eating disorders like obesity or bulimia nervosa.

Persistent poor weight gain is often noted in inborn error in metabolism problem or congenital disorder (usually there are other symptoms of developmental delays associated with this disorder).

Any change in appetite pattern, consider eating disorders, trauma, abuse, or mental health issue.

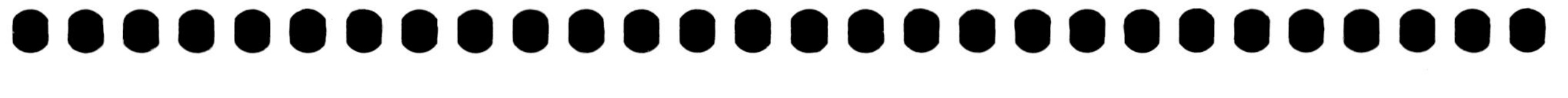

Food Intolerance

Allergies, lactose intolerance especially in people of Latino and African heritage, GERD, inborn error in metabolism, or malabsorption disorder such as celiac disease.

Nausea & Vomiting

Gastroenteritis, intestinal parasites, food intolerance, GERD, pregnancy, appendicitis, intussusception, drug or alcohol toxicity, poisoning, or other environmental toxins. Also consider eating disorder.

Pain

Acute appendicitis, inflammatory bowel disease, irritable bowel syndrome, volvulus, intussusception, hepatitis, ulcer, reflux, abdominal migraine/seizure disorder, trauma, or constipation. Constipation is the most common cause of abdominal pain in children.

Swelling

Organomegaly, constipation, abdominal mass. Wilms tumor, usually presenting as a palpable abdominal mass, is most found in preschoolers.

Stooling Patterns and Appearance

Bloody stools can indicate presence of hemorrhoids, rectal fissure, or inflammatory bowel disease.

Thin ribbon stool usually in Hirschsprung disease.

Persistent bulky, frothy, foamy stool are often associated with cystic fibrosis.

New onset frothy, foul-smelling diarrhea found with Giardia infection or other parasitic infestation.

Constipation without/with diarrhea seepage found in functional constipation and encopresis respectively. Stool seepage without constipation, consider spina bifida occulta.

Urinary:

Frequency, Amount, Odor

Oliguria can indicate renal disease or dehydration.

Polyuria noted in poorly controlled diabetes mellitus, UTI, renal disease.

Urinary urgency without other symptoms is often reported in children with constipation.

Foul odor often indicates infection, dehydration, food effect, i.e., asparagus ingestion.

Bladder Control

Enuresis (wetting after toilet trained) can be related to UTI, familial enuresis, reflux, diabetes, renal disease, or spina bifida occulta. Consider tight clothing in girls. Occasionally related to mental health or behavioral issue.

Reproductive (Female):

Menarche

Record: Onset, regularity, duration, amount, pain, discharge, last menstrual period (LMP).

> With all menstrual problems, pregnancy should be considered as part of the differential diagnosis.
>
> Refer for evaluation with pediatric endocrinology or gyn for primary amenorrhea if no menses by age ≥14 years, especially in the presence of normative puberty findings and for secondary amenorrhea if no menses for 3 months after last period in the absence of pregnancy. Spotting or irregular bleeding between menses can represent normal developmental regulatory problems or indicate pathology such as polyp, cervical disease
>
> Report of mild dysmenorrhea is usually a normative finding; more severe or difficult to treat dysmenorrhea can be associated with pelvic inflammatory disease, endometriosis, other.
>
> Identify premenstrual syndrome (PMS).

Physiologic vaginal discharge should be present. Unusual or excessive vaginal discharge often associated with infection including STI or other problem such as a retained tampon.

Sexual History

Note pain, bleeding, discharge, age at onset of first experience, number of partners, safe sex practices, and birth control methods. Sexual orientation

History of STIs including genital warts. Note the earlier the onset of intercourse and the frequency of partners the greater the risk for endometriosis, cervical cancer, STIs. History of spontaneous or induced abortion; hormonal contraception (pill, patch, ring, implant, IUS) vs. other methods; use of condoms (latex allergy history). Identify risk factors for venous thrombotic event (VTE) with use of systemic hormonal contraceptions including positive family hx VTE, personal history of obesity, tobacco use, others. Remember that some forms of systemic hormonal contraception can interact with other medications, especially certain antiepileptic drugs and impact their efficacy.

History of Sexual Abuse

Increased risk for dysfunctional relationships, difficulty with sex, damage to reproductive organs, depression, posttraumatic stress disorder (PTSD).

Reproductive (Male):

Circumcised or not circumcised male

Discharge

Urethritis, STIs, urethral valve weakness with urine leakage.

Penile Pain

Hygiene problems, balanitis, phimosis, prolonged erection (especially sickle cell crisis response, use of erectile dysfunction medications)

Lesions

Genital warts, genital herpes, scabies, lice

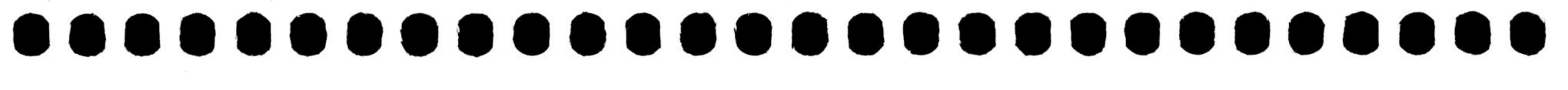

Testicular Pain, Swelling

Torsion, trauma, epididymitis, hernia, tumor, hydrocele, anabolic steroid use.

Sexual History

Identify risk for STIs, safe sex practices, number of partners, sexual orientation

History of Sexual Abuse

Policy Statement: Protecting Adolescents: Ensuring Access to Care and Reporting Sexual Activity and Abuse. Society for Adolescent Medicine. Available at: http://www.aafp.org/about/policies/all/adolescent-protecting.html

Resource for parents and providers available at: http://www.nctsn.org/trauma-types/sexual-abuse

Endocrine:

Precocious Puberty

Early developer, thyroid, pituitary or adrenal disorder in girls, exogenous estrogen intake; boys more likely to have central nervous system (CNS) tumor as cause of early onset puberty. See Quick Reference Chart: *Puberty*.

Delayed-onset Puberty

Describe thyroid, pituitary, hypothalamus, adrenal dysfunction

Short Stature

Constitutional or familial short stature, growth hormone deficiency

Temperature Abnormalities/Imbalance

Newborn instability phenomenon, hypoglycemia, hyperthyroidism, hypothyroidism, frostbite sequelae, Raynaud's disease.

Excessive Thirst, Excessive Urination

Diabetes mellitus, renal disease, dehydration

Failure to Thrive

Inborn errors of metabolism, cystic fibrosis, abuse (organic or non-organic), HIV, malignancy marasmus occurrence increases prior to age 1 year whereas kwashiorkor occurrence increases after 18 months.

Musculoskeletal:

Muscle or Joint Pain

Migratory arthritis secondary to illness syndrome, juvenile rheumatoid arthritis (JRA), strain/sprain, malacia process of the bone, overuse injuries. Hip pain – consider Legg-Calvé-Perthes disease, slipped capital femoral epiphysis (SCFE).

Bone Pain

"Growing" pain, recurrent pain syndrome, stress, trauma, cancer, overuse injuries, fractures

Weakness

Muscular dystrophy, anemia, malnutrition, exhaustion, dehydration, lactic acid accumulation

Swelling

Strain/sprain, nodular formation, fluid accumulation, hemarthrosis

Deformities

Congenital, fractures, juvenile rheumatoid arthritis (JRA), hemophilia response, sickling crisis reaction, clubbing, steroid use, rickets, or scoliosis

Neurological:

Learning

Grade level inequities with age and immaturity increase risk of grade repeating. With learning difficulties consider attention deficit disorder/attention deficit hyperactivity disorder (ADD/ADHD), perceptual learning problems, hearing/language development problems, developmental delay, lead or other environmental toxicity, anemia, sleep deprivation, nutritional deprivations, conduct disorder, thyroid disease, or mental health issue.

APA Practice Guidelines for ADD/ADHD available at:

https://pediatrics.aappublications.org/content/pediatrics/early/2011/10/14/peds.2011-2654.full.pdf

Dizziness

Vertigo, use of select medications, drugs, hypotension, CNS tumor, aspirin (ASA) overdose, or environmental toxin exposure.

Fainting or Blackouts

Substance abuse, syncope, hypoglycemia, hypotension, seizures, tumor, hyperventilation, anoxia, eating disorders, cardiac disorders including hypertropic obstructive cardiomyopathy or long QT syndrome. In adolescent females, consider pregnancy.

Weakness

Muscular dystrophy, multiple sclerosis, failure to thrive (FTT), cardiac disease, diabetes, renal disease, seizures, other progressive neurological disorder

Paralysis

Fractures, trauma, post viral, Guillain Barré syndrome, intracranial bleed, tumor, myasthenia gravis, or Bell's palsy

Hand Dominance Determined before Age 2

Cerebral bleed, post meningeal/encephalitis effect, neurological disorder

Change in Gait

Vertigo, dystrophy, substance abuse, cerebral or spinal tumor

Tremors & Involuntary Movements

Seizure disorder, tics, Tourette syndrome, habits, intracranial lesion, substance abuse effect or withdrawal

Personality Changes

Seizures, anabolic steroid use, substance abuse, prescription or OTC drug use, mental health disorder, intracranial lesion, or effects of physical, mental, emotional abuse.

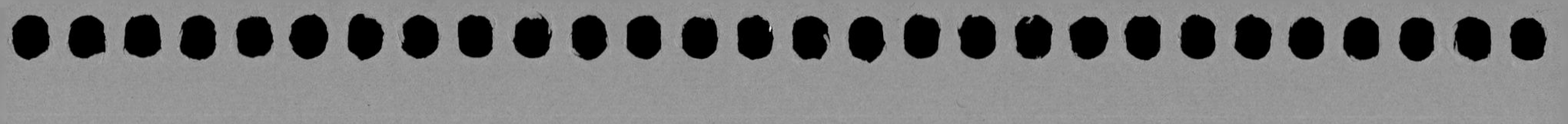

Cue Card Series

Pediatric Physical Assessment

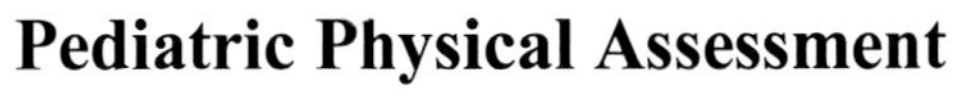

Pediatric Physical Assessment

Table of Contents

I. General Appearance

Examination Principles

Newborn Examination: Areas of Concentration

1. Congenital anomalies
2. Birth injuries
3. Acute neonatal illnesses
4. Determination of gestational age and appropriateness of size for gestational age

Sequence of Newborn Exam

1. General observations
2. Eye examination, presence or absence red reflex bilaterally
3. Auscultation anterior/posterior chest (heart and lungs)
4. Auscultation/palpation of abdomen
5. Palpation of femoral and upper extremity pulses
6. Head-to-toe exam of anterior and posterior body
7. Remaining neurologic assessment

8. Ortolani/Barlow maneuver
9. Moro reflex

Infant Examination: Areas of Concentration

1. Growth (nutrition)
2. Motor development
3. Language development (hearing)
4. Emotional development (temperament, attachment, social interaction, autism)
5. Vision and strabismus screening
6. ≤6 months: Congenital anomalies; delayed sequelae of newborn problems, genetic disorders

Toddler/Preschool Examination: Areas of Concentration

1. Speech clarity and content
2. Gait and appearance of lower extremities
3. Hearing and middle ear status
4. Vision and strabismus screening

5. Emotional and behavioral development: Autonomy and independence, orientation to self and environment
6. Heart murmurs
7. Nutrition
8. Safety
9. Oral health

School-age Child Examination: Areas of Concentration

1. Common minor infections (respiratory, skin)
2. Aches and pains (headaches, stomach aches)
3. Allergic disorders (asthma, eczema, hayfever)
4. Growth and development (nutrition)
5. Scoliosis screening*
6. Pubertal development (if appropriate)
7. Energy and stamina (physical activity)
8. School achievement (mental health, ADHD, bullying, friends)
9. Safety and sport injuries (helmets, concussions)
10. Vision, hearing, and oral health

Adolescent Examination: Areas of Concentration

1. Pubertal development
2. Social and academic competence
3. Nutrition, eating disorders, steroid use
4. Risky behaviors including substance abuse, high risk sexual activity
5. Safety and sports injuries (concussions, sprains/strains, dislocations, overuse)
6. Scoliosis screening*

**Scoliosis screening should be at a minimum done on all girls at both age 10 and 12 (grade 5 and 7) and all boys once at ages 13 or 14 (grade 8 or 9) per AAOS, AAP, SRS, and POSNA consensus guidelines, available at: http://www.aaos.org/uploadedFiles/1122%20Screening%20for%20the%20Early%20Detection%20of%20Idiopathic%20Scoliosis%20in%20Adolescents%202%201%2016.pdf*

Age and Sex: This infant/child/adolescent is a _______ month/year old _________ (sex) who appears to be in __________________ health and developmentally ________________________ for his/her age.

Record any evidence of illness, poor hydration, distress, pain, developmental delay, overall well-being.

Vital Signs: The infant/child/adolescent weighs ________ (pounds/ounces [g/kg]), is ________ (inches [cm]) tall, and head circumference (HC)/occipital frontal circumference (OFC) is _______ (inches [cm]) (until 3 years of age). The child/adolescent's body/bone frame appears __________ (small, medium, large). BMI:________(>2 years of age)

Record physical conditioning and history of family stature/maturation patterns. Record on growth chart.

T: _________ (Fahrenheit, Centigrade, route of recording)

P: _________ (Rate, rhythm, PMI, presence of pulses in all extremities)

R: _________ (Rate, rhythm, evidence of distress)

BP: _________ (Left, right, sitting, standing. Begin routinely at age 3 years)

Note comparison with previous vital sign recordings.

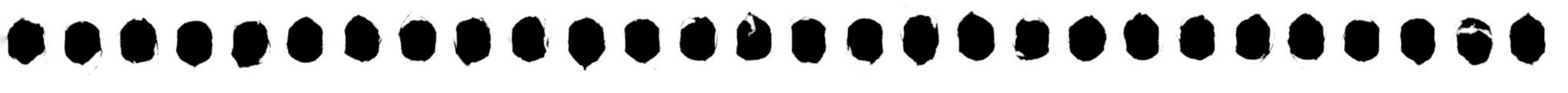

Behavior/Mental Health:

Social interaction is appropriate.

> Early infancy: Record evidence of lack of eye contact, smiling, vocalization, social play, or connection with others.
>
> Toddler: Record orientation to name, joint attention skills, awareness of others, lack of eye contact, alterations in hearing or speech.
>
> Child: Note parent/caregiver-child interactions including caregiver effort to influence child's behavior in exam room. In child, sadness, fear beyond what is typical for age and setting, apathy, hyperactivity

Dress, Appearance, Personal Hygiene: Child/adolescent's dress and hygiene/grooming are appropriate for the weather and setting.

> Record any deviation from above, noting parental and sibling dress, grooming, hygiene.

<u>Facial Expression, Manner, Attention Span, Fine and Gross Motor Activity</u>:
Child/adolescent's expressions and manner are appropriate to the occasion. Child/adolescent pays appropriate attention and was appropriately involved in the exam. Fine and gross motor activity was rhythmic, equal in all extremities, and developmentally appropriate.

Record any deviation from the above, especially in fine and gross motor activity and those things not mentioned under Affect. Record achievement on a structured developmental assessment tool such as Ages and Stages Questionnaire (ASQ) agesandstages.com, Parents' Evaluations of Developmental Status (PEDS) http://www.pedstest.com, or Denver Developmental Screening Test www.developmentalscreening.org/about.htm

<u>Speech</u>: Child/adolescent's speech is developmentally appropriate, spontaneous, smooth, and articulate (as indicated by developmental achievement).

Link to AAP file on screening tests (some listed below), through Bright Futures available at: https://brightfutures.aap.org/Bright%20Futures%20Documents/Developmental_Screening_Tools.pdf

The ELM (Early Language Milestone) scale for children 0–3 years of age;
The CAT (Clinical Adaptive Test)
CLAMS (Clinical Linguistic and Auditory Milestone Scale) for children 0–3 years of age
The Infant Monitoring System for children aged 4–36 months
The Early Screening Inventory for children 3–6 years of age
The Peabody Picture

The primary language in the family is _______________. Child/adolescent speaks _______________as a first language.

> Record any evidence of stuttering, lisping, tongue-thrusting, high-arched palate, tongue-tie, history of ear infections, parental language/speech style, absence of speech, family history for speech problems, hearing status, and school progress/problems.

Cognition: Child/adolescent demonstrates cognitive ability appropriate for his/her age as demonstrated by __________ (school grade, performance, or level of discussion with provider).

> Record evidence of mismatch between grade level and age, significant variation in child/adolescent's understanding of subject under discussion with provider that is not accounted for by English-as-a-second language or development level.

Orientation: Child/adolescent is alert, appropriately oriented to the environment, identifies his/her parent/caregiver, and can answer age-appropriate questions about self, place, time (year, season, date, month, location).

> Record any deviation from above that cannot be explained by cultural, language, or developmental level.

II. Skin

<u>Color, Temperature, Texture, Turgor, Lesions</u>: The child/adolescent's skin is soft, moist, with normal turgor. There is no evidence of hypo/hyperpigmented areas, lesions, birthmarks, masses, or trauma. Describe exactly as visualized using objective physical findings.

> Record evidence, size, number, placement of, changes in Café au lait spots, flat nevi, spider nevi, hemangiomas, salmon patches, vitiligo, Mongolian spots, warts, moles.
>
> Record evidence of rashes, plaques, abrasions/injury, poor skin turgor.
>
> Note timing of onset of rash, part of body where rash first appeared, distribution pattern-clustered, dense, or scattered, if new or recurrent problem, any recent exposure to illness or toxins. Quick Reference Chart: *Acute, Febrile, Rash-producing Illness*.

Assessment Criteria for Hydration Status

Parameter	Mild 3–5%	Moderate 6–9%	Severe >10%
BP	Normal	Normal	Normal to reduced
Pulse quality	Normal	Normal to slightly decreased	Moderately decreased
Heart rate	Normal	Normal to increased	Increased (sometimes bradycardia)
Skin turgor	Normal	Recoil<2 sec	Recoil>2 sec, tenting
Fontanels	Normal	Slightly depressed	Depressed
Mucous membranes	Slightly dry lips, thick saliva	Dry lips and oral mucosa	Very dry lips, oral mucosa

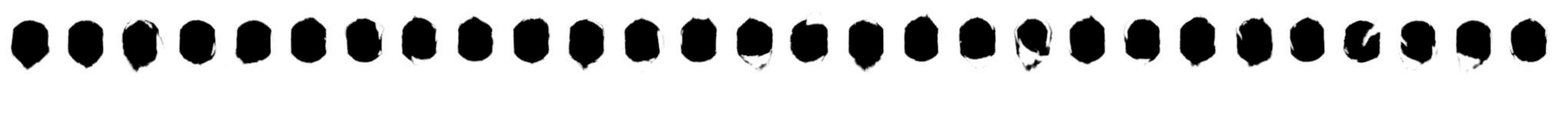

Assessment Criteria for Hydration Status			
Parameter	**Mild 3–5%**	**Moderate 6–9%**	**Severe >10%**
Eyes	Normal, tears present	Slightly sunken, tears decreased	Deeply sunken, tears absent
Capillary refill	Normal (<1.5 seconds)	Delayed (1.5–3 sec)	Delayed (>3 sec)
Mental status	Normal	Normal, fatigued, restless, irritable	Apathetic, lethargic, unconscious
Urine output	Slightly decreased	Decreased	Minimal
Thirst	Normal, to slightly increased	Moderately increased	Very thirsty or too lethargic to assess

CDC Acute Diarrhea Management dehydration evaluation; available at: http://www.cdc.gov/disasters/disease/diarrheaguidelines.html

WHO Acute Diarrhea Management: https://pediatrics.aappublications.org/content/pediatrics/129/5/e1211.full.pdf

Describing Common Primary Skin Lesions

- **Macule**: Flat, ≤ 1 cm, varies in color, well circumscribed, i.e., freckle, flat nevus
- **Papule**: Elevated, circumscribed, ≤ 1 cm, varies in color, i.e., wart, mole, molluscum contagiosum
- **Patch**: Macule that is >1 cm, varies in color, i.e., vitiligo, mongolian spot
- **Plaque**: Raised, solid, circumscribed lesion >1 cm with flat top, varies in color, i.e., psoriasis, eczema, lichen simplex, tinea corporis
- **Pustule**: Elevated, superficial, purulent fluid-filled lesion, size and color vary, often in hair follicle or sweat pore i.e., acne vulgaris
- **Cyst**: Circumscribed, palpable lesion filled with liquid or semi-solid material, color and size vary, i.e., sebaceous cyst, cystic acne
- **Vesicle**: Elevated, circumscribed, ≤ 0.5 cm, fluid-filled lesion, varies in color, i.e., blister, varicella, insect bite, herpes simplex

- **Bulla**: Circumscribed, raised lesion, vesicle ≥1 cm, i.e., large blister, burn, bullous impetigo
- **Nodule**: Elevated, firm palpable lesion within the dermis, <2 cm in diameter, i.e., lipoma, fibroma, erythema nodosum, hemangioma
- **Wheal**: Raised area of edema, pale center, variable in diameter, blanches, varies in color, may be transient, i.e., urticaria, mosquito bites, erythema multiforme
- **Comedo:** Plugged pore, open-blackhead, closed-whitehead, i.e., acne
- **Burrows:** Linear markings, i.e., scabies, mites
- **Telangiectasia**: Fine red lines produced by capillary dilation, i.e., acne rosacea

Describing Common Secondary Skin Lesions (secondary to chronic primary lesion or trauma)

- **Scale**: Flaky, irregular, dry or oily keratinized epidermal lesion, color and size vary, i.e., psoriasis, seborrheic dermatitis, tinea versicolor
- **Crust**: Dried exudate, color and size varies, i.e., impetigo
- **Lichenification**: Rough, thickened, induration of skin with shiny surface secondary to chronic rubbing, i.e., chronic atopic dermatitis
- **Fissure**: Linear crack from epidermis to dermis, usually small and reddened, i.e., athlete's foot (tinea pedis), intertrigo
- **Erosion**: Loss of epidermis (partial or full thickness), usually following rupture of vesicle or enlargement of fissure, i.e., herpetic vesicle, impetigo
- **Ulcer**: Loss of epidermis and dermis, color and size vary, i.e., pressure sore
- **Scar:** Permanent change due to healed damage, i.e., surgery, burn, keloid (hypertrophied healed lesion)

- **Purpura:** Purple macular lesion >1 cm, i.e., Henoch-Schönlein
- **Hematoma:** Collection of blood from ruptured vessels >1 cm, i.e., ecchymosis
- **Petechiae:** Non-blanching pink to purple vascular lesion 1–3 cm, i.e., strep throat
- **Desquamation:** Peeling scales, often in sheets, i.e., strep infection

Configuration of Skin Lesions

- **Annular or circular**: Begins centrally and spreads to the periphery, i.e., ringworm
- **Confluent**: Lesions that run together i.e., hives
- **Discrete**: A single, distinct lesion, i.e., mole
- **Grouped**: Seen in clusters or sets, i.e., herpes
- **Linear**: In a line or stripe, i.e., poison ivy dermatitis
- **Zosteriform**: Lesions along a dermatome or nerve root, i.e., herpes zoster
- **Nummular:** Coin-shaped, localized in a limited area, i.e., eczema

Nails: Nail beds are intact, appropriately colored, with good capillary refill (<3 seconds). Nail plates are smooth without evidence of "nail-biting." Cuticles are white.

> Record clubbing, thickening (fungal infection), thinning (systemic/ chronic disease, respiratory, cardiac, malnutrition, anemia), or evidence pus or erythema (inflamed paronychia). Also note artificial nails or polish. Blue color (cyanotic disease)

Source:

Habif, T. (2012) Dermatology DDxDeck, 2nd Edition, St. Louis, MO: Elsevier Health Sciences.

Habif, T. (2011) Skin Disease, 3rd Edition, St. Louis, MO: Elsevier Health Sciences.

III. Head

Skull/Scalp: The size of the skull is developmentally appropriate and is in proportion to the rest of the body. HC/OFC is________. The anterior fontanelle is _____________ (open/closed), is _______ (normal [flat or slightly inward], sunken, bulging) and is approximately _________cm in size. The posterior fontanelle is _____________ (open/closed), is _______(normal [flat or slightly inward], sunken, bulging) and is approximately ______cm in size. There is no overriding of the suture lines, the skull feels round, smooth without evidence of gross deformities or tenderness. The scalp is free of lesions, infestations, scaling, flaking. Note head control and movement.

> Fontanelles: Anterior closed by 9–18 months, posterior closed by 4 months.

Record any deviations in the above especially noting early/late closure of the fontanelles, whether normal (flat, or slightly inward), sunken (dehydration), or bulging (increased intracranial pressure)*, craniostenosis, genetic condition, macro/microcephaly, hydrocephaly, craniotabes, caput succedaneum, cephalhematoma (fracture often present underneath), abrasions. Persistent head lag or tilt, indicate hypotonia, congenital torticollis.

*Remember to assess fontanels when the infant is calm and upright. Fontanels may appear to be bulging in a crying infant or one who is lying in a supine position

Record evidence of parasitic, fungal, eczematous/seborrheic lesions, alopecia.

Facial Structures: *Have child/adolescent smile, laugh, frown, relax face. If crying, observe facial movements.* Facial structures move symmetrically and are midline. There is no evidence of drooping, asymmetry, or disproportionate features.

Record alterations in the above noting palsy, ptosis, tics, facial hemangiomas, facial evidence of chromosomal anomalies, frontal bossing or fetal alcohol syndrome, malalignment of structures.

Hair: Hair is evenly distributed, healthy, and without evidence of easy plucked or hair loss. The color is __________.

Record any breakage of hair shafts, areas of hair loss, poor hygiene, thinning, use of hair dyes, loss of luster. Note cultural considerations, hair care products

IV. Eyes

Red Flags: Eyes that flutter from side to side or up and down or cross
Eyes always watery or very sensitive to light
Any white, grayish-white, or yellow colored material in the pupil
Any change in the eyes appearance
Persistent redness of the eye or pus
Frequent rubbing eyes or squinting
Any drooping or bulging of eye
Frequent tilting or turning of head instead of eyes

Lids, Lid Margins, Eyelashes, Lacrimal Duct: Lids evident bilaterally and close in unison with blinking to cover entire eye. The lid margins are appropriately colored without evidence of lesions, edema, ptosis, inversion, or eversion. The eyelashes are appropriate formed and evenly distributed without evidence of flakiness, scaling, or parasitic infestation. Eyebrows symmetrical.

Record abnormalities in the: Palpebral fissure (space between upper and lower lid that can be increased in exophthalmus or decreased in severe dehydration), presence of blepharitis (eyelid inflammation), hordeolum (sty/localized infection of lid), chalazion (retention cyst within lid margin), ptosis (drooping of lid present in myasthenia gravis, damage to CN III, damage to sympathetic nerve as in Horner syndrome), nits (pubic or head lice), seborrhea of lid, lacrimal duct stenosis (chronic tearing from one eye or palpable mass below medial canthal tendon), dacryocystitis (infection of lacrimal duct), or incomplete closure of eyelid (hyperthyroidism).

Conjunctiva/Sclera: Bulbar and palpebral conjunctiva and sclerae are appropriately and uniformly colored bilaterally without injection, discharge, or lesions.

In darker-skinned individuals, there are often small dots of pigment near limbus as well as a slight scleral uniform yellowing.

Conjunctivitis (chemical, allergic, bacterial, viral irritation, injection, discharge), injury, dermoid cyst, pterygium (opaque triangular shaped lesion extending from nasal/lacrimal area across cornea), icteric sclerae.

Cornea and Iris: Corneas are smooth, transparent, with equal light reflex noted in both eyes and no evidence of esotropia or exotropia. There is no evidence of scarring, lesions, or opacities. Iris is intact with uniform pigmentation.

> Coloboma (failed embryonic fusion anywhere from optic disc to iris, usually associated with a systemic syndrome), or aniridia (absence of iris). Albinism (absence of color in iris).
>
> White or grayish/brown flecks (Brushfield spots) present in peripheral iris in >75% of children with Trisomy 21 (Down syndrome).

Pupils: Pupils appropriately constrict and dilate bilaterally to direct and consensual light. Note when accommodate.

Funduscopic: The red (or ethnicity appropriate) reflex is present bilaterally. The lens is clear without opacities. The vessels of the retina appear normal and there is no evidence of papilledema.

Absence or incomplete red reflex or opacity of lens can indicate a cataract, retinoblastoma, or congenital glaucoma in children. In children with darker skin tone, the "red" reflex often has a more orange tone. Papilledema indicates increased intracranial pressure. Presence of retinal hemorrhage suggestive of shaken-baby syndrome.

Extraocular Movements (EOM): *Have the child/adolescent follow the pen or light, without moving their head, in the 6 cardinal positions. Pause in the extreme lateral and upward gaze to observe for unusual nystagmus. Conduct a cover test which evaluates alignment as young as 4 months.*

EOMs are intact without evidence of nystagmus or strabismus.

Variation in the position of the eyes from the normal position, demonstrating either esotropia, exotropia, or floating position.

Untreated strabismus can lead to amblyopia (loss of vision). Congenital nystagmus can be associated with Down syndrome, seizures, abnormalities of optic nerve in older children may be drug overdose or chemical toxicity.

Visual Acuity and Color Blindness: *Use Allen near cards, ages 2–3 years, Snellen Tumbling E 3–5 years and a standardized Snellen chart for older children for visual acuity test.*

20/20 not possible until 6–8 years of age.

Refer to eye care specialist with visual acuity of:

- *20/50 or less at age 3 years*
- *20/40 or less at age 4 years.*

Use the Ishihara plates to test for color blindness in older children,

Hardy-Rand-Rittler (HRR) in younger children (performed usually between ages 4–8 years).

Visual acuity is _____ (OD), _________ (OS), _______ (OU) (corrected or uncorrected). There is no evidence of color blindness.

Myopia occurs in school-age children as eye matures, most often in girls ages 9–11 years with boys slightly older, increases with age.

Visual Fields: Visual fields are intact by confrontation.

V. Ears

<u>Auricles</u>: Are appropriately formed, symmetrical, in appropriate alignment with the outer canthus of the eye; appropriately shaped without lesions, skin tags, masses, deformities, discharge, erythema, crustiness, or pain.

> Malposition (low set) can indicate a congenital syndrome with renal anomalies or chromosomal abnormality; skin tags may be associated with hearing loss or sinus track infections; pain and discharge can indicate an otitis externa or infected pierced ear.

<u>Mastoid</u>: Non-tender, no redness, or swelling.

> Abnormality may indicate mastoiditis secondary to otitis media.

<u>Ear Canal</u>: *In a younger child gently pull canal down, and back, and in older child/adolescent gently pull ear upward and back.*

The ear canals are patent bilaterally without evidence of discharge, lesions, or foreign bodies. There is a ________ amount of cerumen present in the canal.

Describe texture of cerumen – moist, dry. Indicate if TM fully or partially visible or if cerumen fully obstructs view of TM.

Source: The American Academy of Otolaryngology – Head and Neck Surgery Foundation (AAO-HNSF) Clinical Practice Guideline: Cerumen Impaction, available at http://oto.sagepub.com/content/139/3_suppl_1/S1.full.pdf+html

Lack of patency can indicate a structural abnormality, hearing loss. Discharge may be indicative of softened or liquid cerumen, purulent drainage secondary to ruptured tympanic membrane (TM), infective response to foreign body, "swimmer's" ear (otitis externa).

Tympanic Membrane: Pearly gray and shiny with bony landmarks clearly visible, concave, and no evidence of injection, erythema, perforation, retraction. Bright light reflex is visible and within normal limits. Membranes move under insufflation.

A variation in TM possibly indicates serous otitis/otitis media with effusion, secondary effect from fluid in ear, acute otitis media, or eustachian tube dysfunction.

Diagnosis of acute otitis media (AOM) includes loss of TM anatomic landmarks, distortion or loss of cone of light, increased TM vascularity or generalized erythema, bulging, loss of mobility on insufflation coupled with otalgia or other symptoms consistent with AOM.

Otitis media with effusion (OME) findings include retraction or fullness of TM without erythema; air bubbles or yellowish fluid present behind TM often couples with impaired TM mobility.

Ear infections are more frequent in younger children. Risk factors include age, which gender, passive smoking, bottle-feeding. Approximately 40–60% of otitis media (OM) are viral in origin and resolve without antimicrobial therapy. If child is asymptomatic, hold the use of antibiotics. AAP criteria for managing otitis media and otitis with effusion available at: http://pediatrics.aappublications.org/content/131/3/e964

Auditory Acuity: *Most states have implemented universal hearing screens in infancy (Evoked Otoacoustic Emission Testing [EOAE], Automated Auditory Brainstem Response [ABR], or Brainstem Auditory Evoked Response [BAER]) and audiometry in school years. Behavioral observed Audiometry and Impedance diagnostic testing is used in most pediatric practices. Should be able to hear in both ears 500−6000 frequency (Hz) at 25 decibels (db).*

Note startle reflex present in newborns, note language development in toddlers/preschoolers with a language screen such as Early Language Milestone Scale (ELMS), have children over 3 years old cover an ear and you whisper a word in the uncovered ear at a distance of approximately 1−2 feet (0.3−0.6 m). Repeat on other side. For younger children, while child is distracted, create a noise and look for child's response to finding what made the noise or finding where noise is coming from.

Weber test: *Usually not conducted until school-age years. Place a vibrating tuning fork midline on top of patient's head and ask the patient to identify where the sound is heard – left, right, or both ears.*

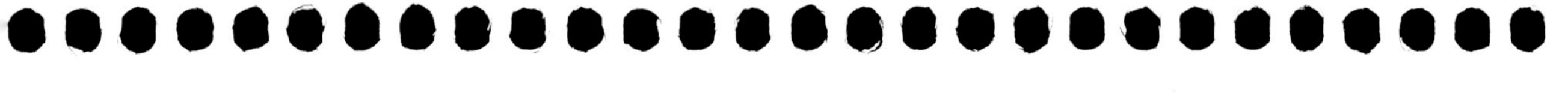

Weber is intact without lateralization.

> Lateralization to impaired ear indicates conductive hearing loss.
> Lateralization to unimpaired ear suggests sensorineural hearing loss.

Rinne test: *Place a vibrating tuning fork on patient's mastoid, ask child/adolescent to tell you when the vibration stops. Once it is no longer audible, place the tuning fork in front of the ear and ask the child/adolescent if it is still audible.*

Rinne is intact with air conduction (AC) > than bone conduction (BC).

> Deafness or impaired hearing–2 major types:
>
> 1. Conductive hearing loss: Caused by a mechanical interruption of sound waves from external ear to inner ear. Most often occurs with acute otitis media and usually persists for up to 3 months post infection. Usually resolves without special intervention. When persistent, occasionally corrected through surgical intervention (tympanostomy tubes). Hearing aids rarely used. Conductive hearing loss when severe can result in BC>AC.

2. Sensorineural hearing loss: Caused by inability of the inner ear or nerve to respond to sound waves. Often not helped by hearing aids. Causes 90% of all serious, profound, persistent hearing loss. Sensorineural hearing loss is AC>BC in conjunction with abnormal Weber test and whisper test.

Etiology for sensorineural hearing loss includes heredity, encephalitis, intrauterine infections, prolonged/repeated exposure to loud noise, use of select medications, prematurity, severe jaundice or hemorrhage, also associated with many syndromes

Mixed conductive and sensory loss is also possible.

VI. Nose and Sinuses

<u>Nose</u>: Is midline without obvious deformities and deviations

<u>Nares</u>: Are patent bilaterally *(in newborn gently occlude each nostril, keep mouth closed and watch for nasal movement with respirations to rule out choanal atresia).*

<u>Nasal Septum, Turbinates, and Mucosa</u>: Are intact, midline, normal size and color (pink), moist without ulceration, swelling, erythema discharge, or polyps.

> Deviated septum increases potential for sinusitis. Ulcerated/perforated septum often secondary to sniffing or snorting illicit substances. Enlarged turbinates usually indicative of inflammatory reaction (allergic, viral, infection). Erythema of turbinates and mucosa indicate viral or bacterial infection while bogginess usually related to allergies. Clear rhinorrhea found in allergies and viral infections; purulent rhinorrhea present in viral or bacterial infections. Malodorous mucopurulent discharge from one nostril, consider foreign body or sinusitis.

> Epistaxis, nasal hemorrhage often associated with irritation, allergy or trauma. A transverse crease across nose (allergic salute) often associated with recurrent nasal itch or discharge.

<u>Sinuses</u>: Frontal and maxillary sinuses are non-tender bilaterally, without fullness, erythema, or discoloration. (Sinus development)

Palpate and percuss these sinus areas to observe for tenderness.

> Post-nasal drip, cobblestone appearance on back of throat, sinus tenderness, warmth, color. Note color of nasal discharge, length of time and time of day for nasal congestion and cough. Halitosis is often indicative of bacterial sinusitis, pharyngitis, or dental disease.

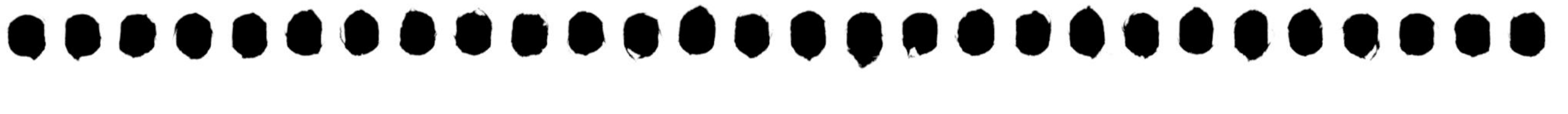

VII. Mouth

Lips: Are intact, uniform and symmetrical, pink, moist, without evidence of lesions, ulcerations, cracking.

> Lesions often seen with herpes simplex (vesicles and crusts) or impetigo (pustules and crusts), cracking from dryness, malnutrition, cleft lip, or chronically enlarged tonsils or adenoids. Color change can indicate anemia (cyanosis – bluish tinge).

Tongue: Is moist, pink, straight, midline, and freely movable without evidence of exudates, pitting or dermographia, discoloration, nodules, lesions.

> Impaired mobility is possibly related to "tongue-tied" (also known as ankyloglossia, can cause poor suck and later speech impairment); dermographic tongues are normal but become more pronounced with illness states; discolored tongues can be inherited or related to illness; deviation of tongue possibly indicative of abnormality of CN XII resulting in inability to nurse or bottle-feed. Painless oral lesions can be cancerous from chewing tobacco use; also consider syphilitic chancre.

<u>Mucosa and Gingiva</u>: Healthy appearance, color consistent with ethnicity, firm, moist without lesions, masses, coating, or bleeding

> Abnormalities possibly related to anemia (color), dehydration (moisture), lesions (Coxsackie/herpes virus), coating (illness state or candida), stress or poor oral hygiene.

<u>Hard and Soft Palate</u>: Are intact, patent without lesions.

> High arch or other abnormalities indicative of cleft palate; Epstein pearls in the newborn, Koplik spots (rubeola), petechiae (strep throat). Infant, yellow color hard palate indicates jaundice. Asymmetrical rise in soft palate indicates abnormality CN X.

<u>Uvula</u>: Midline without evidence of ulcers, erythema, deviation, or clefts.

> Abnormalities such as redness, enlargement and/or exudate suggest Coxsackie virus, or bacterial infection. Contralateral uvula deviation noted in peritonsillar abscess. With bifid uvula, look for possible high cleft palate.

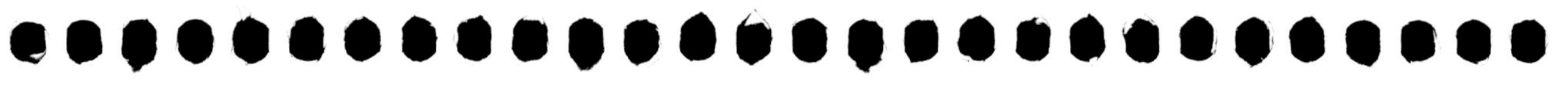

Tonsils: Present bilaterally without evidence of injection, swelling, exudate, or asymmetry.

> Not usually visible in infants until 2 years of age, peak size at age 2–6 years.
>
> Abnormalities commonly include acute hypertrophy and erythema with or without exudate, possibly indicative of viral or bacterial infection. Asymmetric hypertrophy associated with painful swallowing, trismus (pain with opening jaw) with contralateral uvula deviation suggestive of peritonsillar abscess. Pitting or enlarged crypts can be due to recurrent infections or chronic allergies.

Pharynx: Healthy without evidence of lesions, erythema, edema, or post-nasal discharge. Intact gag reflex.

Dentition: Number of primary teeth _____, secondary teeth _____. Appearance is white without evidence of dental caries, white spots or plaque, appropriate alignment.

Dental abnormalities can be related to staining from fluoride use or intrauterine exposure to select antibiotics (tetracyclines), chronic illness states; early childhood caries/bottle-mouth syndrome. Malalignment, malocclusion usually not corrected until age 8 or 9 years when more permanent teeth are visible and jaw development is more mature. Natal teeth often associate with cleft palate, neonatal teeth (teeth erupt within first month) often associated with precocious puberty. Delayed eruption of primary teeth associated with Down syndrome, hypothyroidism, and endocrine disorders. White spots indicate demineralization of primary teeth. Surface wearing can be seen with bruxism. Erosions at gum line often present with recurrent vomiting, induced or involuntary.

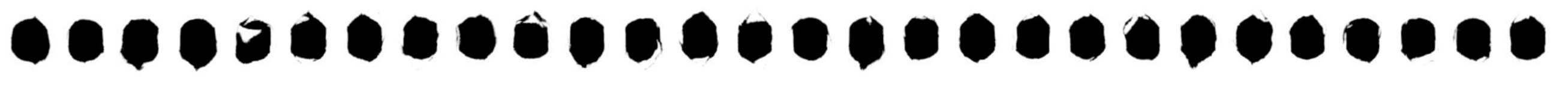

VIII. Nodes

Non-palpable and non-tender, size___________

<u>Location</u>: *Preauricular, postauricular, occipital, tonsillar, submaxillary, submental, superficial cervical, posterior cervical, deep cervical, supraclavicular, epitrochlear, axillary, mesenteric, inguinal, popliteal.*

> Note presence, placement, size, tenderness, associated symptoms, length of time nodes enlarged, pain upon palpation, local or generalized. Lymphadenopathy when acute is often infective states (viral or bacterial). With persistent, nontender lymphadenopathy, consider malignancy.

IX. Neck

Note shape, symmetry, pain, or irritability.

Mobility: Full range of motion.

> Restrictions in range of motion can be seen in torticollis, cervical strain or mass, adenitis, lymphadenopathy. Shortened neck or masses, webbing can be indicative of Turner syndrome, cystic hygroma.

Trachea: Midline without deviation.

> Abnormality may be related to thyroid or other cystic mass, mediastinal shift from pneumothorax or cardiac tamponade.

Thyroid: Palpable and appropriate size for age without evidence of masses, tenderness, thyromegaly.

> Abnormalities in size may be goiter (generalized enlargement), thyroid nodule (localized enlargement), autoimmune response as seen in Graves' disease or Hashimoto thyroiditis.

X. Thorax and Lungs

Chest Wall: Exhibits normal structure without evidence of curvature or protrusion.

> Abnormalities may indicate congenital structural anomalies that may interfere with respiratory effort, i.e., pectus carinatum, pectus excavatum, or scoliosis; or nutritional deficits, i.e., rickets. Barrel chest associated with cystic fibrosis.

Respiratory Rate, Rhythm, Effort: Regular, non-labored with a rate of ________________ per minute appropriate for age.

> Note respiratory distress (use of intercostal muscles, nasal flaring, audible wheezing, grunting), tachypnea (can indicate cardiac disease, pneumothorax, consolidated mass). Prolonged inspiratory phase often noted with upper airway obstruction as in croup with prolonged expiratory phase evident in lower airway obstruction like asthma. Apnea >15 seconds and accompanied by central cyanosis, presence of Cheyne Stokes breathing require immediate evaluation and intervention.

Note rapidity of onset of symptoms. Inhalation anthrax is characterized as rapid onset of respiratory distress and failure within 24 hours of the onset of flu-like symptoms without rhinorrhea. Clinical presentation of pneumonic plague includes fever, cough, dyspnea, bloody/watery, and purulent sputum.

Percussion: Findings indicate resonance throughout lung fields

Abnormalities in percussion often include dullness, indicative of increased density as in pneumonia, pleural effusion, or hyperresonance suggesting decreased tissue perfusion and air trapping as noted in asthma, cystic fibrosis, bronchopulmonary dysplasia (BPD), pneumothorax. Percussion often deferred when evaluating infants and young children.

Auscultation: Bronchovesicular sounds heard bilaterally throughout lung fields.

Vesicular breath sounds are soft, low-pitched heard over most of lung fields, heard upon inspiration > expiration; bronchial breath sounds are higher-pitched, arising from bronchi and heard over bronchus and trachea, inspiration < expiration; bronchovesicular breath sounds are loud, high-pitched heard anteriorly at 1st and 2nd ICS, posteriorly between scapula and bronchial tree, may be heard equally inspiration or expiration.

> Stridor is a high-pitched, loud inspiratory sound heard with upper airway obstruction, edema, croup, or foreign body ingestion (FBI). Grunting–low-pitched expiratory sounds, due to partial closing of glottis and attempt to generate greater airway pressure. Snoring, rough snorting sound, either expiration or inspiration is often noted in upper respiratory infection (URI), nasal polyps, hypertrophy of adenoids or tonsils. See Quick Reference Chart: *Differential Diagnosis of Stridor in Children*.

Crackles (rales), found in lower lung fields, represent the sound of air going through small, fluid- or exudate-filled airways, and can be indicative of pneumonia, heart failure (HF), bronchopulmonary dysplasia, or cystic fibrosis.

Wheezing sound of air going through a narrowed airway and is usually present initially on expiration (difficulty getting air out) or inspiration (difficulty getting air in). Noted in lower airway disease such as in asthma, bronchiolitis, bronchitis, pneumonia, HF, cystic fibrosis, inhaled foreign body.

Rubs are a rubbing or grating sound heard during inspiration and expiration caused by the movement of two inflamed surfaces. They are evidence of pleurisy.

Egophony, Bronchophony, Whispered Pectoriloquy:

If there is concern about consolidation, these tests can be done.

Egophony: Over the area of consolidation, the spoken "e" will sound like an "o."

Bronchophony: Over an area of consolidation, spoken words increase in clarity.

Pectoriloquy: Over the area of consolidation, whispered words will increase in clarity.

XI. Breasts

Female and Male:

> Neonatal breasts are often engorged (male and female) due to maternal estrogen; this usually regresses within a few weeks without intervention. Note presence or absence of supramammary nipples without other signs of puberty that can regress spontaneously.

Female: *Inspect full adult breast with child/adolescent sitting with hands on hips and then with them stretched above head, then lying down with hands behind head. With pendulous breasts have child/adolescent stand and lean forward. Preferred position for examining developing breasts; have child/adolescent supine with arm under head. Examine the following:*

Shape, Symmetry, Size: The breasts are symmetrical, smooth, convex, and ________ in size. Color is consistent with skin tone without evidence of lesions, masses, dimpling, retractions, discharge, or striae.

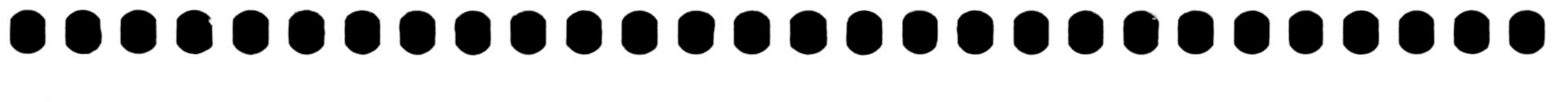

Thelarche, beginning of breast development first sign of puberty, is signaled with breast budding. Breast asymmetry is a common normal variant in adolescence.

Areola Size, Shape, Location: Areola is __________cm in diameter, round, appropriately centered without evidence of lesions, scaling, erythema, or tenderness.

Nipple Appearance: Nipples are _________ (inward or outward) pointing without deviation or discharge.

Palpation: There are no masses, tenderness, lesions/nodes palpable on breast, areola, nipple, or axillary region.

> Abnormalities revealed by palpation can be as a result of fibroadenoma (most common reason for breast mass in adolescents), proliferative breast disease (AKA fibrocystic disease, cysts <1 cm, frequently mobile), physiological swelling and tenderness during menstrual cycle, or, rarely, malignancy. Atrophy due to eating disorders, macromastia due to obesity. Wide-set nipples are found in a variety of genetically-based conditions including Turner syndrome, Down syndrome, Edward syndrome, others.

Male: Symmetrical without masses, budding, tenderness, or lesions.

Adolescent benign gynecomastia (usually disappears in 2 years after pubertal onset) or obesity-related gynecomastia (usually disappears after weight loss, also known as pseudogynecomastia). Gynecomastia can also be noted with select drug use including marijuana, corticosteroids, atypical antipsychotics, and spironolactone.

Breast cancer in males is rare, especially in presence of family history of early onset (premenopausal) breast cancer or family history of breast cancers in males.

XII. Heart

BP: Is ______________, equal on both arms, lower leg. (Take at every visit, focused and comprehensive, starting at age 3 years)

Pocket guide from NHLBI/NIH of BP Measurement available at:
www.nhlbi.nih.gov/health/public/heart/hbp/bp_child_pocket/bp_child_pocket.pdf

O_2 saturation______ (if indicated)

Precordium: *The palmar surface of the hand is most sensitive to vibratory sensation while the 2nd–3rd fingers are most sensitive to pulsation.*

There are no pulsations, lifts, taps, or heaves in the aortic, pulmonic, tricuspid, or mitral regions.

> Thrill is a vibratory sensation caused by turbulent blood flow and felt with grade ≥ IV heart murmurs found with aortic or mitral valve disease or congenital cyanotic heart disease states. Best felt with fingertips.

Point of Maximum Impulse (PMI): Apical pulse is present at apex, 4th–5th ICS, midclavicular line.

> Displaced apical pulse is evident in cardiomegaly or dextroposition of the heart, or mediastinal shift, and/or ventricular overload.

Rate and Rhythm: The rate is ________ beats per minute (BPM) and regular appropriate for age.

Heart Sounds:

> Listen for evidence that S1, S2 are present without splitting, murmurs, rubs, nor is there evidence of S3 or S4. Assessments should be done at rest, supine and standing, and after 5 minutes of running in place. Use both diaphragm and bell.

***S1** represents events surrounding the closure of mitral and tricuspid valves, heard best at 5th ICS midclavicular and left sternal border. A split S1 usually normal in young children, although can be noted in the presence of right bundle branch block.*

***S2** represents events surrounding the closure of aortic and pulmonic valves heard best at 2nd ICS on left and right of sternal borders. Physiologic split S2 heart sound is often heard in adolescents, with an increase in the split on inspiration. However, the presence of a fixed or loud S2 indicates an abnormality such as hypertrophic cardiomyopathy, aortic stenosis, uncorrected aortic or ventricular septal defect.*

***Physiologic S3** is a result of rapid filling left ventricle in children and changes/diminishes when position changes from lying to sitting.*

***Pathologic S3** is indicative of systolic dysfunction and is most often noted in the presence of heart failure.*

***S4** is indicative of diastolic dysfunction and is most often noted in hypertrophic cardiomyopathy recurrent myocardial ischemia and/or poorly controlled HTN.*

***Ejection clicks:** Extra heart sounds between S1 and S2 suggest bivalvular abnormality.*

> Record evidence of lack of change of splits, rate, rhythm with position change or after exercise.

Murmurs: There are no murmurs present.

Murmurs represent the sound of turbulent blood flow and collision currents
Physiological or innocent murmurs: *Occur in 30–50% of all children. Found in systole, ejection, heard best over LLSB, and usually a Grade II or III.*

Still murmurs: Soft, medium-pitched, early-mid systolic, musical/vibratory, heard best at apex and left sternal border in lying position and diminishes with sitting. Present anytime in infancy–adolescence, usually 2–7 years of age. More common in children with thin chest wall.

Venous hum: Continuous humming sound heard best at infraclavicular and supraclavicular areas while sitting (diminishes when lying down or turning head). Present in ages 3–6 years; a benign finding.

Hemic murmur: A benign, transient systolic murmur noted in the presence of fever, anemia, exercise, pregnancy and heard best in aortic/pulmonic region. Disappears when the underlying condition is resolved.

Pathological murmurs: *Those found in diastole and systole and usually a grade II–III or higher.* Diastolic murmurs are always pathologic

Pathologic murmurs are a result of acquired or congenital heart defect states.

When performing the cardiac exam, you might find it helpful to close your eyes during auscultation while listening so you can focus solely on the heart sounds. If you are having difficulty distinguishing systole from diastole, keep in mind that the S1 heart sound marks the beginning of systole and is heard virtually simultaneously with the carotic upstroke. If a murmur or other abnormal heart sound is heard, you might find it helpful to tap out the rhythm with your thumb and index finger with your eyes closed and "feel" in which finger the abnormal sound is heard.

If murmur is heard, describe the following:

Intensity:

Grade I: Very faint, barely audible

Grade II: Soft, quiet but easily heard

Grade III: Moderately loud without a thrill (usually same intensity as the normal heart sounds)

<u>Grade IV</u>: Loud and associated with a thrill (the sensation of turbulent blood flow) and possible lift/heave

<u>Grade V</u>: Very loud, associated with thrill and lift

<u>Grade VI</u>: Often heard without a stethoscope and associated with thrill and lift.

Timing:

Systole or diastole or both

Early, mid, late, throughout systole or diastole

Location of where murmur heard loudest

Tone as high- or low-pitched, buzzing, musical, blowing, harsh, heard best with bell (low-pitch) or diaphragm (higher-pitch)

Radiation: Presence or absence, state location– neck, axilla, infraclavicular or supraclavicular space, scapula

Provoking positioning: Change in murmur provoked by supine, sitting, standing, and/or squatting; holding breath.

Long QT syndrome: *Familial predisposition, usually triggered by significant exercise (i.e., swimming, running, etc.). Most common presentation is post-exertion syncope with 50% reporting symptoms by age 12 years. Often report exercise- or stress-induced chest pain.*

The use of select medications including certain atypical antipsychotics can induce QT prolongation. See https://crediblemeds.org/ for additional information. Confirm diagnosis with electrocardiogram.

Cardiac abnormalities associated with genetic conditions− Down syndrome, Marfan syndrome, connective tissue disorders. Signs of cardiac problems include hypercyanotic spells, sweating, squatting, assuming knee-chest position. Must rule out breath holding spells.

Infants and young children with L to R shunts− hx frequent respiratory infections, failure to thrive, ↑rest periods, ↓activity

Acute cardiac problems may present with sudden fever ≥5 days, strawberry tongue, conjunctivitis, edema eyelids, erythema of palms and soles of feet, ↑lymph nodes, rash, likely indicative of Kawasaki disease

Marfan Stigmata (skeletal, cardiovascular, ocular):

Tall, thin
Arm span > height
Arched palate, crowded teeth
Arachnodactyly (long, thin fingers)
Pectus excavatum or carinatum (sunken or pigeon chest)
Scoliosis
Flat feet
Hyper-flexible joints
Severe myopia (near sightedness)
Stretch marks without history of weight gain/pregnancy
Murmurs (aortic aneurysms, dissection, mitral valve prolapse)

If positive findings: Deny clearance for sports until evaluation, which can include ECG, echocardiogram, chest CT or MRI

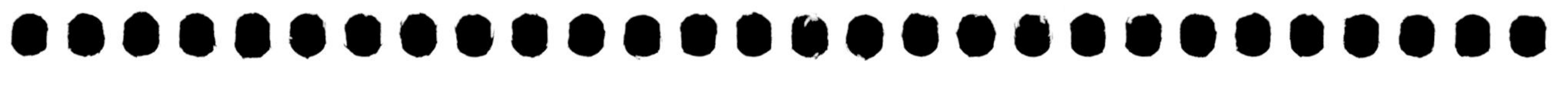

XIII. Peripheral Vascular

Pulses: Presence and equality of the following pulses: *(Note deviations and rate on a scale from absent [0] to 4+.)* No palpitations, syncope, or chest pain.

Temporal _____ Popliteal ___

Brachial _____ Posterior tibialis _____

Radial _____ Dorsalis pedis _____

Femoral _____

Absence of pulses or inequality of BP may indicate aortic coarctation, slow capillary refill indicative of poor perfusion. Irregularity due to dysrhythmia.

If diminished femoral pulses, obtain cardiac echocardiogram and/or chest CT to evaluate for aortic coarctation

Edema: None present.

Varicosities: None present.

Combined hormonal contraceptive use (pill, patch, ring) can exacerbate varicose vein-related symptoms such as leg heaviness but their presence is not a contraindication to the use of systemic hormonal contraception.

Syncope:

Weakness may have preceding pallor and dizziness, falling, quick recovery, loss of consciousness, usually benign but may indicate cardiac, neurological or metabolic disorder, rule out breathholding in younger children, especially toddlers, hyperventilation in adolescents.

Chest Pain:

Most often costochondritis in older children, adolescents, sharp well localized pain, reproduced with pressure, often following recent viral illness or exercise. ECG indicated.

XIV. Abdomen

<u>Umbilicus</u>: No drainage, infection (in infants), no hernia or masses

<u>Abdominal Contour and Color</u>: Flat, symmetrical without scars, striae, spider nevi, masses, bulging. (Children <4 years old have normal potbelly appearance)

> Presence of increased abdominal girth can indicate Wilms' tumor *(do not palpate if Wilms' tumor is suspected)*, Hirschsprung disease (usually in newborn who has not passed stool in first 24–48 h of life), constipation, stool, pyloric "olive" like mass (pyloric stenosis), organomegaly (hepatic and/or splenic enlargement), ascites, distended bladder, diaphragmatic hernia (neonate), or intestinal obstruction. Often accompanied by palpable abdominal mass.

<u>Bowel Sounds</u>: Present in all 4 quadrants.

Auscultate bowel sounds before palpation so as not to create bowel sounds and miss a "silent" abdomen.

Note intensity, frequency of bowel sounds.

> Hypoactive or absent bowel sounds in infant can be noted in paralytic ileus, obstruction. Hyperactive may be diarrhea or mechanical obstruction; with bowel obstruction, a "tinkling" sound is occasionally noted.

Palpate: There are no masses, tenderness, organomegaly, or hernia. No evidence of abnormality in the flank areas. Liver is palpable 1–2 cm below costal margin in infant through young school-age.

Children are often ticklish and if you have them help you palpate, they have less resistive reactions. Begin palpation in lower abdominal quadrants and work your way upward.

> Presence of masses can be indicative of tumor, Wilms' tumor, Hirschsprung disease (usually in newborn who has not passed stool in first 24–48 h of life), stool, pyloric "olive" like mass (pyloric stenosis), organomegaly (hepatic and/or splenic enlargement), bladder, polycystic kidneys, ascites, high-riding rib cage with falsely perceived enlargement of organs.

Tenderness often noted in appendicitis, mesenteric adenitis, inflammatory bowel disease, gastroenteritis, constipation, other intestinal disorders, or PID.

Presence of rebound tenderness suggests peritoneal irritation or inflammation as in appendicitis or other acute intraabdominal problem.

Organ tenderness can be indicative of acute or chronic hepatitis, mononucleosis, sickle cell anemia with or without crisis, malaria (those recently arriving from or traveling in high-risk areas).

Percussion: Tympani throughout except over liver and splenic regions where appropriate dullness is present. No costovertebral (CVA) tenderness.

CVA tenderness suggestive of pyelonephritis. Abdominal tenderness may indicate an intraabdominal problem or organ inflammatory/irritation process.

Acute abdominal pain: *In pubescent girls, pelvic inflammatory disease and appendicitis have similar presentations. As a result, the workup should include CT scan, pregnancy test, and pelvic exam. In males, rule out hernia, epididymitis.*

XV. Genital/Rectal

Female: External genitalia normal female, intact, appropriately developed for age, no evidence of discharge, lesions, or trauma. Urethra present and midline. Clitoris present and vaginal opening apparent. Pubic hair distribution (if pubescent) is normal.

Female newborns and infants, check patent vaginal orifice, may have normally enlarged labia majora, clitoris, dull labia minora 2° maternal estrogen in the neonatal period. Not uncommon to note creamy or blood-tinged vaginal discharge also.

Adrenarche: Development of pubic and axillary hair

See Tanner staging at: http://healthvermont.gov/family/toolkit/tools%5CJ-1%20CARD%20Tanner%20Stages.pdf

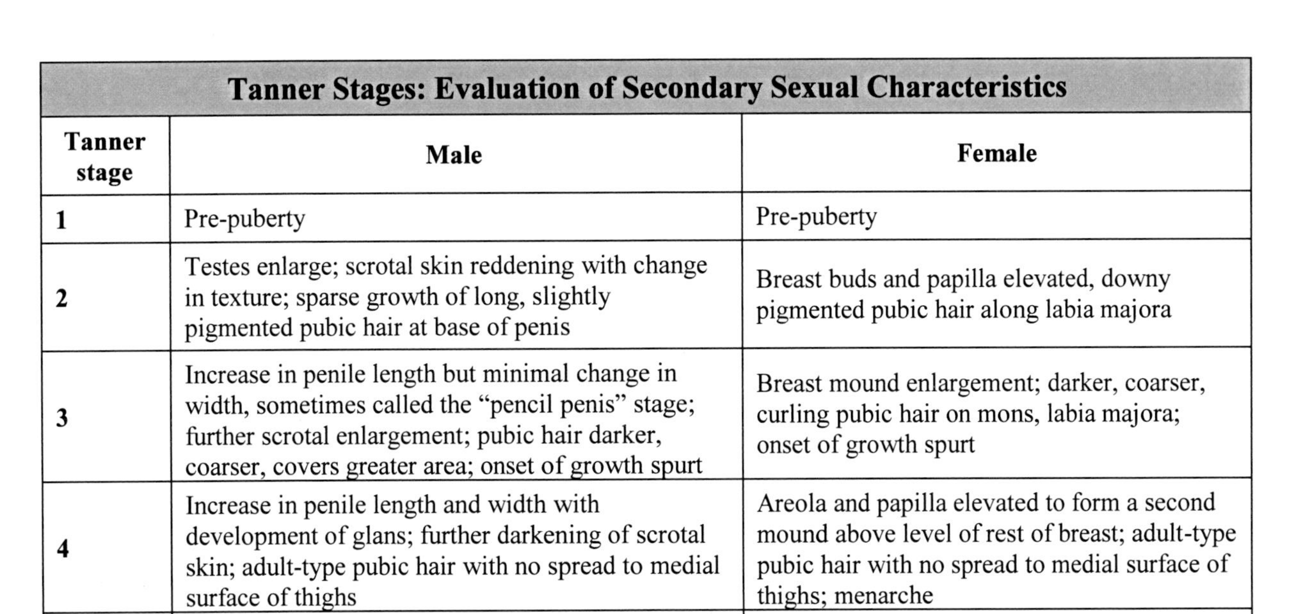

Tanner Stages: Evaluation of Secondary Sexual Characteristics		
Tanner stage	**Male**	**Female**
1	Pre-puberty	Pre-puberty
2	Testes enlarge; scrotal skin reddening with change in texture; sparse growth of long, slightly pigmented pubic hair at base of penis	Breast buds and papilla elevated, downy pigmented pubic hair along labia majora
3	Increase in penile length but minimal change in width, sometimes called the "pencil penis" stage; further scrotal enlargement; pubic hair darker, coarser, covers greater area; onset of growth spurt	Breast mound enlargement; darker, coarser, curling pubic hair on mons, labia majora; onset of growth spurt
4	Increase in penile length and width with development of glans; further darkening of scrotal skin; adult-type pubic hair with no spread to medial surface of thighs	Areola and papilla elevated to form a second mound above level of rest of breast; adult-type pubic hair with no spread to medial surface of thighs; menarche
5	Full adult genitalia; adult-type pubic hair with spread to medial surface of thighs, possibly	Recession of areola to mound of breast, extension of pubic hair to medial thigh

Source: Duderstadt, K. (2013) Pediatric Physical Examination, 2nd Edition, St. Louis, MO: Elsevier Health Sciences

> Evidence of abuse i.e., genital warts, vaginitis, requires careful history, behavioral observations, documentation, initiate protocol for further evaluation and forensic exam which may warrant photographs.
>
> Questionable or ambiguous genitalia need investigation for adrenal hyperplasia disease, sexual agenesis disorders, or intersex condition.
>
> Hymenal irregularities or absence could be acute or chronic trauma.

Pelvic Exam: If appropriate *(for specific vaginal or pelvic complaints or those with suspected sexual abuse, and routinely at age 21 years).Offer STI testing with all sexually active teens. Be sure to use speculum size appropriate for child's age and virginal status.*

Vaginal canal is healthy, appropriately colored without evidence of trauma or discharge.

> Abnormalities may indicate sexual abuse. With sexual agenesis, vaginal opening is absent. Vaginitis may also indicate STIs, diabetes, bacterial infection. Also consider foreign body ingestion (FBI), hygiene.

Cervix is appropriately colored without evidence of lesions, trauma, discharge, tenderness.

> Cervical motion tenderness is present in pelvic inflammatory disease (PID) or if traumatized. Abnormal vaginal discharge is often present with STIs.
>
> Common for females to have teaspoon or so of odorless, clear to yellow discharge 6 months prior to the onset of menarche

Uterus is appropriate size, shape, position without tenderness or masses.

> Enlarged uterus may indicate pregnancy (most common reason in teenage females), fibroids, or tumor.

Adnexal region is without tenderness or masses.

> Mass or tenderness can suggest tubal (ectopic) pregnancy, abscess (as part of PID), ovarian cyst, or tumor.

Male: Penis is normal male, circumcised/uncircumcised (prepuce or foreskin should be fully retractable after age 3 in uncircumcised males), urethral opening midline, appropriate size for age. Testes are descended bilaterally without masses or tenderness. No hernias present. No penile discharge. If pubescent, pubic hair evenly distributed. *Examine supine position for infants/young children, standing in adolescents.*

> Phimosis: Delayed separation of foreskin after 5 years of age.
>
> Paraphimosis: Retracted foreskin that cannot be reduced (*Emergent)*
>
> Hypospadia is the urethral opening underneath the glans penis while epispadia is opening on top of glans. Bladder abnormality common cofinding with urethral abnormality. Consider ambiguous genitalia
>
> Cryptorchidism: Absence of testes or retractible in inguinal canal, refer for surgical evaluation ↑risk testicular cancer in adolescence.
>
> Hydrocele (a painless transilluminating enlargement of scrotum, caused by fluid accumulation) not uncommon in newborns and are usually spontaneously reabsorbed within the first year of life.

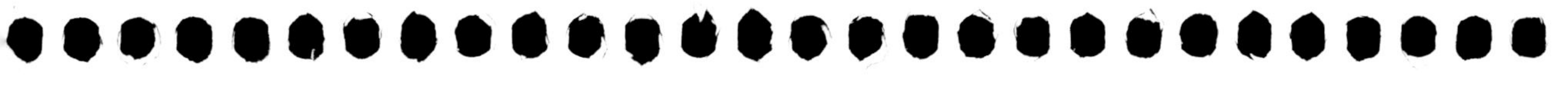

Communicating (risk of hernia) vs. non-communicating hydrocele

Swelling in scrotum enlarges during day or when sitting and reduces when supine consistent with communicating hydrocele

Testicular torsion seen in school-age boys (Prehn's sign negative, high risk for those with repaired infantile hernias and those in high contact sports). Presents with acute pain, swelling, redness of involved testes – surgical emergency. Epididymitis often presents with the same symptoms usually requiring supportive treatment and antibiotics.

Hypogonadism found in chromosomal anomalies: Klinefelter syndrome, ↑risk prostate cancer if treated with testosterone in adolescence

Large gonads noted with puberty in Fragile-X syndrome males.

Hernia: Inguinal mass or protrusion of tissue. If easily reducible, may observe, if not, refer for surgical evaluation.

Ambiguous genitalia usually associated with genetically-based conditions.

Male and Female:

Rectal: External mucosae are appropriately colored with no lesions or evidence of trauma present. Sphincter patent and intact, no evidence of fissures, skin tags, bleeding, hemorrhoids, or dimpling; in infants note patent anus.

> Abnormalities such as bruising, redness, swelling, discharge or external trauma may indicate sexual abuse (also examine oral cavity); functional constipation response, Crohn's disease.
>
> Dimpling and discoloration of anus may be due to metal toxin ingestion.

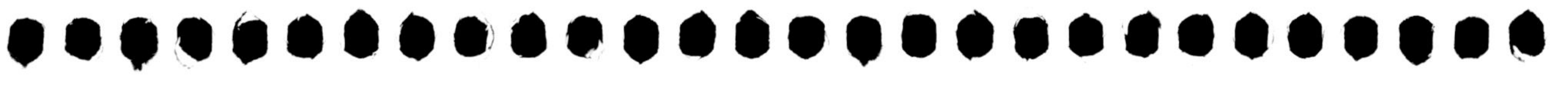

XVI. Musculoskeletal

No extra digits or abnormalities. All joints have full range of motion without tenderness, nodules, swelling, erythema, crepitus, deformities. All muscles demonstrate equal strength and are well developed. Normal gait, posture and symmetrically proportionate extremities.

> Polydactyly: Supernumerary digits. Syndactyly: Webbed or fused extremities. Both indicative of genetic condition or developmental delay.
>
> Positive history at risk for sports: Any family history sudden death from cardiovascular problem <50 years of age; history of chest pain, dyspnea, syncope, palpitations, loss of consciousness, fainting, previous concussion.
>
> Female Athlete Triad– anorexia, amenorrhea, and osteopenia.
>
> Childhood RA– symmetrical joint redness. Swelling, pain

Range of Motion:

Temporomandibular Joint: Open and close without catching, clicking, pain

<u>Cervical Spine</u>: Flexion of chin to chest, extension of head back, lateral bending with ear touching corresponding shoulder, rotation with chin touching corresponding shoulder

<u>Shoulders</u>: Abduction *(arms out to each side level with shoulders)*, adduction *(cross arms in front)*, extension *(arms straight and behind back)*, flexion *(arms straight and raised over head)*, internal *(hands behind small of back)* and external *(hands behind the neck)* rotation

<u>Elbows</u>: Flexion *(bend arm upward)*, extension *(straighten arm)*, supination *(turn palms upward)*, pronation *(turn palms down)*

<u>Wrists</u>: Flexion *(bend wrist down)*, extension *(bend wrist up)*, ulnar deviation *(laterally deviate wrist)*, radial deviation *(medially deviate wrist)*

<u>Hands/Fingers</u>: Flexion *(make a fist)*, extension *(straighten fingers)*, abduction *(spread fingers)*, adduction *(bring fingers together)*

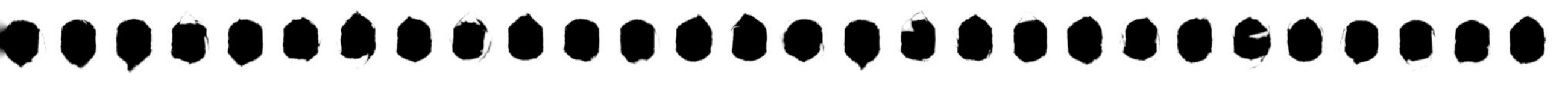

Hips: Flexion *(bring knee toward body in flexed and straight position)*, extension *(straighten leg)*, abduction *(move leg laterally)*, adduction *(move leg medially across center of body)*, internal and external rotation *(turn leg medially and laterally), in newborn do the Ortolani and Barlow tests to evaluate for developmental dysplasia of hips*

Ortolani maneuver: Hip flexed 90 ° – one leg at a time. Thigh is gently abducted, bringing femoral head interiorly. If congenital hip reduces into acetabulum it will make a palpable and audible "clunk," which is a positive test.

Barlow maneuver: Hip is flexed to 90 ° – one leg at time. Thigh is gently adducted and pushed posterior towards exam table. If hip dislocates the examiner will feel the head dislocate out of the acetabulum. This is less sensitive than Ortolani. If Barlow maneuver is positive, confirm with Ortolani maneuver.

Knees: Extension and flexion

Ankles: Plantar flexion *(point toes toward floor)*, dorsiflexion *(point toes toward body)*, inversion *(deviate ankles medially)*, eversion *(deviate ankles laterally)*

Feet/Toes: Inversion, eversion, flexion, extension

Spine: Flexion, extension, lateral bending, lateral rotation

> Abnormalities in range of motion often indicates cerebral palsy, dystrophies, electrolyte imbalances, injury, congenital anomalies, scoliosis, developmental dysplasia of hip, slipped femoral capital epiphysis, Legg-Calvé-Perthes disease, femoral anteversion, Osgood Schlatter, metatarsus adductus, equinovarus, pes planus, or clubfoot.

Developmental issues which usually resolve with continued growth and development include genu varum, bowlegged until 2 ½–3 years, knock kneed (Genu valgum) until 7–8 years; tibial torsion until 3–4 years.

Structure: Bones are straight without evidence of calcifications, old fractures, other deformities, pain.

Palpate all bones.

> Abnormalities are occasionally evidence of abuse, osteogenesis imperfecta, cancer, rickets, TB of the bones.

Assess Spinal Straightness: *Perform forward bend test to assess level of shoulders, scapula, hips are equal bilaterally in standing and bending position.* Spine feels in proper alignment in standing and bending position. Note any rotation >5−7 degrees.

> Abnormality in alignment indicative of scoliosis or shoulder malalignment from book bags, briefcases, hand dominance. Referral needed to rule out scoliosis and need for bracing or surgery. Boys at greater risk for needing surgical correction with poorer prognosis for correction. Abnormality occasionally indicates a leg-length discrepancy that is corrected with lifts in shoes.

Strength: Equal in all extremities, *use Oxford scale rating 0−5 ranging from no strength to full strength, for example written as 3/5*

> Abnormalities may indicate dystrophy, tumor, or neurological disorder.

XVII. Neurological

Refer back to the head measurements, presence/absence of fontanelles, other findings on head exam.

> Presence of abnormalities has relevance to neurological problems in younger children.

Structured Developmental Screen: Appropriate for age, see screening section.

> Abnormalities may indicate neurological problems in fine motor, gross motor, speech/language, socialization, and cognitive arenas.

Cranial Nerves: Intact and successfully responsive.

CN I: Olfactory. *No formal test for newborns used. May pass strong smelling substance under infant's nose and observe for startle.*

CN II: Optic. *Assessed by age-appropriate visual acuity screens and visual field ability.*

CN III: Oculomotor. *Assessed by pupillary reactions/size/shape, symmetry of lid closure, and extraocular movements in the 6 cardinal fields of gaze*

> Ptosis indicates possible CN III dysfunction.

CN IV: Trochlear. *Assessed by extraocular movements in the 6 cardinal fields of gaze*

CN V: Trigeminal. *Assessed by facial sensation through light touch and motor ability in ophthalmic, mandibular, maxillary regions and by clenching teeth and blink reflex*

> Tic douloureux (trigeminal neuralgia) and masseter muscle weakness present in myasthenia gravis.

CN VI: Abducens. *Assessed by extraocular movements, specifically lateral movements*

CN VII: Facial. *Assessed by observing infant crying or having child/adolescent smile, frown, resist examiner's opening closed eyes, puff out cheeks, raise eyebrows, show upper and lower teeth.*

> Bell's palsy and sequelae to forceps delivery, when forceps has been across cheeks, is caused by CN VII paralysis.

CN VIII: Acoustic. *Assessed by auditory evaluation with whisper, Weber, Rinne tests. Universal screening for infant hearing required most states, formal audiometry and impedance testing in children.* *See screening section.*

> Abnormalities may be related to tumor or select drug affect.

CN IX & X: Glossopharyngeal and Vagus. *Assessed by speech abilities, tongue extension processed, uvula position and movement, gag reflex with tongue blade.*

CN XI: Spinal accessory. *Assessed through ROM and muscle strength tests for shoulders and neck. Turn infants head, have child/adolescent shrug shoulders.*

CN XII: Hypoglossal. *Assessed by symmetry of tongue. Infant-assess sucking and swallowing; have child/adolescent stick out tongue.*

Motor:

Gait smooth, coordinated, and appropriate for age without evidence of tremors, spasticity, athetoid movements, or atrophy.

No tics, tremors, clonus.

Muscle tone and strength (Modified Ashworth Scale 0–4 scale, no increase in tone – rigidity of affected part).

> Abnormalities may suggest cerebral palsy, muscular dystrophy, cranial or spinal tumor. Tics may indicate Tourette syndrome.

Heel-Toe/Shin Ambulation appropriate for age without evidence of ataxia.

> Abnormality suggests neurological immaturity, tumor, cerebral palsy, dystrophy.

Pronator Drift is absent. *Have child/adolescent stand with eyes closed, feet together, arms extended with palms upward and watch for slow fall and a concurrent pronation of one of the arms/hands.*

> Positive drift indicates neurological immaturity or a spinal tract lesion.

Equilibrium and Coordination

Romberg test *assessed by having the child/adolescent stand, feet together, eyes closed, arms at sides and monitor for swaying.*

Rapid alternation of movements *assessed by having child/adolescent pronate and supinate hands as fast as possible on the legs.*

Finger to nose.

> Positive Romberg and abnormal alternating test indicates neurological immaturity or cerebellar disease. However, consider the age of the child for his/her neurological maturation level.

Deep Tendon Reflexes: Are equal, present, and about a +2 – 3 in all extremities (*Rate both left and right reflexes, use 0–4 scale).*

	Left	Right
Biceps	_______	_______
Triceps	_______	_______
Brachioradialis	_______	_______
Patellar	_______	_______
Ankle	_______	_______

Abnormal reflexes can be indicative of cerebral or spinal problem, endocrine problem, electrolyte problem, especially calcium, magnesium or potassium abnormalities.

XVII. Neurological

Neonatal Reflexes

Symmetrical, most should diminish by 3–4 months and disappear by 4–6 months unless otherwise stated.

	Present	**Absent**	**Brief Description**
Blink			Flash light, blinks eyes
Sucking			Touch mouth, sucks
Rooting			Stroke cheek, turns toward source and sucks
Palmar			Place object in palm, grasps, weakens at 3 months, disappears 12 months
Tonic neck			Place supine, turns head to right, makes fists, disappears 2 months.
Stepping			Hold upright with feet touching ground, walk gait demonstrated
Moro			Loud noise, startles

	Present	Absent	Brief Description
Babinski			Stroke sole of foot, toes fan out, foot curls in, disappears 9−12 months

Mental Status: *Refer back to findings in general appearance section and identify if mental status is healthy, intact, and appropriate for age.* Note level of awareness and orientation.

If indicated perform:

Mini-Mental Status Exam. Available at, www.minimental.com

Modified Glasgow Coma Scale for Infants and Children. Available at http://emedicine.medscape.com/article/2058902-overview

Sports Concussion Guidelines from CDC with specific information to coaches, parents, athletes, and providers regarding preventing and diagnosing TBI/concussions. Available at: http://www.cdc.gov/headsup/youthsports/index.html

Cognitive Ability: *Identify speech and language development, developmental milestone achievement, grade level, thinking processes, comprehension ability, and school success.*

Sensory Function: *Assess sensitivity to pain, temperature, touch.*

XVIII. Children of International Adoption

Before Arrival of Patient to Office:

Review medical records and available history, specifically any pregnancy history or psychosocial history. Clarify existing diagnoses. Review any videos or photographs. Obtain pre-adoption consultation documents.

Determine need to obtain further information.

Review typical health issues to be assessed.

Identify available support systems.

Initial Visit:

- *Review growth and development, history with adoptive parents*
- *Complete head-to-toe physical exam*
- *Conduct routine screening tests*
- *Review existing records. Update immunizations using CDC and ACIP standards and guidelines available at, www.cdc.gov/vaccines/parents/adoptions.html*

- *Generally recommended screening (refer to Red Book for most current recommendations at http://redbook.solutions.aap.org/)*

  Metabolic screen

  CBC with differential, platelet and indices

  Lead level

  Urinalysis

  Screening for hepatitis A, B, C status

  Tuberculin testing despite any previous BCG vaccination, if positive obtain CXR

  Serological test for syphilis

  Stool for O & P × 3, Giardia antigen

  Establish HIV-1, HIV-2 status

  Thyroid function

  Hgb electrophoresis (Especially if Asian, Latino, African ancestry)

  G6PD (Especially if Asian, Latino, Mediterranean, African ancestry)

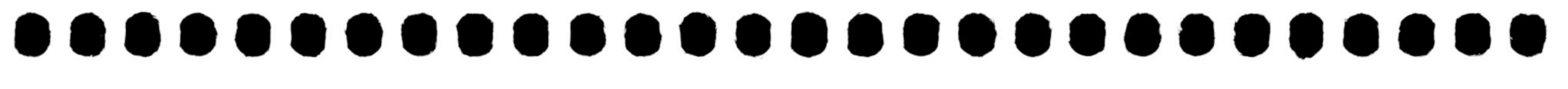

Malaria (In children from tropics, sub-Sahara tropical, Africa, or FUO)

Rickets (Assess vitamin D status, consider x-ray)

Lactose intolerance (Especially if Africa, Latino, Mediterranean, Asian ancestry, consider hydrogen breath test to confirm condition)

Hearing, dental, and vision screening

Structured developmental and mental health screen

Behavioral/developmental and mental health issues, i.e., developmental delay, posttraumatic stress disorder, reactive attachment.

Screen/immunize contacts per recommendation of the Red Book

Guidelines from AAP for International Adoption resource is available at: http://www2.aap.org/sections/adoption/PDF/InternationalAdoption.pdf

Managing Elevated Blood Lead Levels Among Young Children: Recommendations from the Advisory Committee on Childhood Lead Poisoning Prevention (ACCLP)	
0–4 μg/dL (0–0.435 μmol/L)	No significant lead exposure; Educational intervention to avoid exposure
Recommendations of the ACCLP/CDC is to indicate ≥5 to 14 μg/dL (0.24–0.68 μmol/L) at risk	Lead education: Dietary, environmental Follow-up blood lead monitoring
15–19 μg/dL (0.725–0.918 μmol/L)	Lead education: Dietary, environmental Follow-up blood lead monitoring. Proceed according to actions for 20–44 μg/dL (0.966–2.125 μmol/L) if: A follow-up BLL is in this range at least 3 months after initial venous test **or** BLLs increase

Managing Elevated Blood Lead Levels Among Young Children: Recommendations from the Advisory Committee on Childhood Lead Poisoning Prevention (ACCLP) (continued)	
20−44 ug/dL (0.966−2.125 µmol/L)	Lead education: Dietary, environmental Follow-up blood lead monitoring; complete history and physical exam Lab work: Hemoglobin or hematocrit, iron status Environmental investigation, lead hazard reduction, neuro-developmental monitoring Abdominal x-ray, (if particulate lead ingestion is suspected) with bowel decontamination if indicated
45−69 ug/dL (2.17−3.33 µmol/L)	Lead education: Dietary, environmental Follow-up blood lead monitoring, complete history and physical exam Lab work: Hemoglobin or hematocrit, iron status, FEP or ZPP Environmental investigation, lead hazard reduction Neuro-developmental monitoring Abdominal x-ray with bowel decontamination if indicated chelation therapy
≥70 ug/dL (3.38 µmol/L)	Hospitalize and commence chelation therapy Proceed according to actions for 45−69 µg/dL (2.17−3.33 µmol/L)

Source: Summary of Recommendations for Children with Confirmed (Venous) Elevated Blood Lead Levels at www.cdc.gov/nceh/lead/; ACCLP: http://www.cdc.gov/nceh/lead/ACCLPP/acclpp_main.htm

Early Childhood Growth					
Age	**Approx. daily weight gain (g)**	**Approx. monthly weight gain**	**Linear growth**	**Head circum-ference (cm/mo.)**	**Kcal/ kg/day**
0–3 mo.	30	2 lb (0.91 kg)	1.38 inches/mo (3.5 cm/mo)	2	115
3–6 mo.	20	1.25 lb (0.57 kg)	0.79 inches/mo (2 cm/mo)	1	110
6–9 mo.	15	1 lb (0.45 kg)	0.59 inches/mo (1.5 cm/mo)	0.5	100
9–12 mo.	12	13 oz (0.37 kg)	0.47 inches/mo (1.2 cm/mo)	0.5	100
1–3 yr	8	8 oz (0.23 kg)	0.39 inches/mo (1 cm/mo)	0.25	100
4–6 yr	6	6 oz (0.17 kg)	1.18 inches/yr (3 cm/yr)	1 cm/yr	90–100

Source: www.cdc.gov/growthcharts/clinical_charts.htm

Anticipated Early Childhood Developmental Milestones Modified from www.cdc.gov/ncbddd/actearly/milestones/index.html and www.dbpeds.org		
Age	**Motor, reflex**	**Social-interpersonal**
Newborn	• Moves all extremities • Reacts to sound by blinking, turning • Well-developed sense of smell • Preference for higher-pitched voices • Reflexes • Tonic neck • Palmar grasp • Babinski response • Rooting awake and sleep • Suck	• Able to be calmed by feeding, cuddling • Responds to cries of other neonates • Reinforces presence of developmental tasks seen in exam room

Anticipated Early Childhood Developmental Milestones (continued)		
Age	**Motor, reflex**	**Social-interpersonal**
1–2 months	• Lifts head • Hold head erect • Follows objects through visual field • Moro reflex fading	• Spontaneous smile • Recognizes parents
3–5 months	• Reaches for objects • Brings objects to mouth • Raspberry sound • Sits with support • Rolls back to side	• Laughs • Recognizes food by sight
6–8 months	• Sits briefly without support • Scoops small object with rake grip; some thumb use • Hand-to-hand transfer	• Recognizes “No”

Anticipated Early Childhood Developmental Milestones (continued)		
Age	**Motor, reflex**	**Social-interpersonal**
9–11 months	• Stands alone • Imitates peek-a-boo • Picks up small object with thumb and index finger • Cruises	• Follows simple command such as "Come here."
12–15 months	• Walks solo • Neat pincher grasp • Place cube in cup • Tower of two bricks • Scribbles spontaneously	• Indicates wants by pointing • Hands over objects on request
15–20 months	• Points to several body parts • Uses a spoon with little spilling • Walks up and down steps with help	• Understands two-step commands • Feeds self • Seats self in chair • Carries and hugs doll

Anticipated Early Childhood Developmental Milestones (continued)		
Age	**Motor, reflex**	**Social-interpersonal**
24 months	• Kicks ball upon request • Jumps with both feet • Developing handedness • Copies vertical and horizontal line	• Washes and dries hands • Parallel play
30 months	• Walks backwards • Hops on one foot • Copies circle	• Gives first and last name
36 months	• Holds crayons with fingers • Walks down stairs alternating steps • Rides tricycle • Copies circles	• Dresses with supervision

Anticipated Early Childhood Developmental Milestones (continued)		
Age	**Motor, reflex**	**Social-interpersonal**
3–4 years	• Responds to command to place object in, on or under a table • Draws circle when one is shown	• Takes off jacket and shoes • Washes and dries face • Cooperative play • Knows gender
4–5 years	• Runs and turns while maintaining balance • Stands on 1 foot for at least 10 seconds • Counts to 4 • Draws a person without torso • Copies + by imitation	• Buttons clothes • Dresses self except tying shoes • Can play without adult input for about 30 minutes • Verbalizes activities to do when cold, hungry, tired
5–6 years	• Catches ball • Knows age • Knows right from left hand • Draws person with 6–8 parts including torso	• Able to complete simple chores • Sense of gender • Identifies best friend • Likes teacher

Anticipated Early Childhood Developmental Milestones (continued)

Age	Motor, reflex	Social-interpersonal
6–7 years	• Copies triangle • Draws person with at least 12 parts • Prints name • Reads multiple single syllable words • Counts to 30 or beyond	• Ties shoe laces • Generally plays well with peers • No significant behavioral problems in school • Names intended career
7–8 years	• Copies a diamond • Able to read simple sentences • Draws person with at least 16 parts	• Ties shoes • Knows day of the week
8–9 years	• Able to add, subtract, borrow, carry	• Understands concept of working as a team • Able to give response to question such as what to do if an object is accidentally broken

Language Milestones	
Age	**Achievement**
1–6 months	Coos in response to voice
6–9 months	Babbles
10–11 months	Imitates sounds, nonspecific mama, papa
12 months	Specific mama, papa, 2–3 syllable words imitated
13–15 months	4–7 words, jargon, <20% speech understood by strangers

Language Milestones (continued)

Age	Achievement
16–18 months	Extensive jargon, 20–25% speech understood by strangers
19–21 months	20 words, 50% speech understood by strangers
22–24 months	>50 words, 2-word phrases, less jargon, 60–70% of speech understood by strangers
2–2 ½ years	≥400 words, 2–3 word phrases, uses pronouns, ~75% speech understood by strangers
3–4 years	3–6 word sentences, asks questions, tells stories, nearly all speech understood by strangers

Language Milestones (continued)	
Age	**Achievement**
4–5 years	6–8 word sentences, names 4 colors, counts 10 objects correctly

Source: Evaluation and management of the child with speech delay @ http://www.aafp.org/afp/1999/0601/p3121.html also visit www.asha.org

Developmental "Red Flags" In the Young Child

Persistent presence of ≥1 of the indicators warrants further evaluation.

- **By 6 months:** No big smiles or other warm, joyful expressions
- **By 9 months:** No back-and-forth sharing of sounds, smiles, or other facial expressions
- **By 12 months:** Lack of response to name, no babbling or "baby talk," and/or no back-and-forth gestures, such as pointing, showing, reaching, or waving
- **By 16 months:** No spoken words
- **By 24 months:** No meaningful two-word phrases that don't involve imitating or repeating

Source: Modified Checklist for Autism in Toddlers (M-CHAT), available at: http://www.firstsigns.org/downloads/m-chat.PDF

Puberty		
Gender	**Age range at onset of Tanner 2 changes (earliest pubertal changes)**	**Alterations in puberty: Early or late onset**
Female	7 y (thelarche only, earliest breast development) 8 y (pubarche, earliest pubic hair development)–13 y	<7–8 y: Idiopathic in majority (≥85%). Most common puberty disorder. Continuous GnRH agonist analog an option to delay progress, requires specialty evaluation for treatment. >13 y: Multiple factors: Nutrition (low weight), hormonal, genetic (Turner syndrome [XO female]), others
Male	9–14 y	<9 y: Idiopathic in <40% (CNS tumors most often implicated) >14 y: Multiple factors: Nutritional, hormonal, genetic, others

Immunization (IZ) Reaction			
Immunization	**Common reaction (≥25%)**	**Less common reaction (<25%)**	**Rare reaction (< 10^3 to 10^6)**
Anthrax	Soreness, redness, itching at site, myalgia, arthralgia, headache	Fatigue, chills, nausea	Allergic reaction to IZ (rare)
DTaP (diphtheria, tetanus, acellular pertussis)	Soreness, erythema at injection site	Fatigue, poor appetite, GI upset	Seizure, nonstop crying, T≥105°F (41°C), anaphylactic reaction
Haemophilus influenzae type B (Hib)	Erythema at injection site	Fever	
Hepatitis A	Soreness at injection site	Headache, poor appetite	Allergic reaction to IZ (rare)
Hepatitis B	Soreness at injection site	Mild fever	Allergic reaction to IZ (rare)
Inactivated polio virus (IPV)	Soreness at injection site	None reported	None reported
Injectable influenza vaccine (all types)	Soreness, redness at injection site	Aches, mild fever	Allergic reaction to IZ (rare)

Immunization (IZ) Reaction (continued)			
Immunization	**Common reaction (≥25%)**	**Less common reaction (<25%)**	**Rare reaction (< 10^3 to 10^6)**
Live, attenuated virus influenza vaccine via nasal spray (LAIV, FluMist®)	Transient nasal congestion and discharge, headache; harmless virus shed from nose for 3–10 d post-administration	Fever, vomiting, abdominal pain, myalgias	Allergic reaction to IZ (rare)
Measles, mumps, rubella (MMR)	Fever, arthralgia (1 in 4 adult women who receive vaccine)	Mild rash, lymphadenopathy	Seizure, allergic reaction (rare), potential though not proven teratogen
Meningococcus types A, C, Y, W-135 (Menactra®)	Erythema at injection site	Fever	No serious adverse effects noted
Pneumococcal conjugate vaccine 13 (PCV13, Prevnar®)	Erythema at injection site, T ≥100.4ºF (38ºC), usually in children only	Fussiness, loss of appetite (up to 80%, lasts up to 24–48 h) in children only	None noted to date
Pneumococcal polysaccharide vaccine (Pneumovax®)	Erythema at injection site	Fever, myalgia	Allergic reaction to IZ (rare)

Immunization (IZ) Reaction (continued)			
Immunization	**Common reaction (≥25%)**	**Less common reaction (<25%)**	**Rare reaction (< 10^3 to 10^6)**
Quadrivalent human papillomavirus, ([Types 6, 11, 16, 18] vaccine [Gardasil®]), bivalent HPV ([Types 16, 18] vaccine [Cervarix®])	Soreness, swelling, erythema at injection site	Generalized body aches, mild fever, headache (1 in 3)	Serious reactions rare (<0.3%) Reports of post-IZ fainting (sitting or supine position for 15 mins post-IZ recommended)
Rotavirus, live, oral, pentavalent vaccine (RotaTeq®) (pediatric only)	Fussiness, fever on day of immunization	Short-term GI upset (diarrhea, less often vomiting)	Serious reactions rare. No observed increase in rate of intussusception
Serogroup B Meningococcal (MenB®)	Soreness, swelling, erythema at injection site, mild generalized malaise	Fainting	Allergic reaction to IZ (rare)

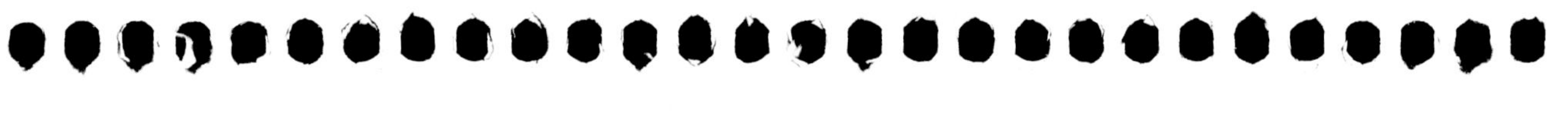

Immunization (IZ) Reaction (continued)			
Immunization	**Common reaction (≥25%)**	**Less common reaction (<25%)**	**Rare reaction (< 10^3 to 10^6)**
Smallpox (live vaccinia virus vaccine) (special use only)	Vaccine delivery results in weeping lesion that contains live vaccinia virus	Fatigue, headache, myalgia, regional lymphadenopathy, lymphangitis, pruritus, and edema at vaccination site	Viral replication, shedding occurs at vaccination site. Unintended transmission possible immediately after vaccination until scab separates from the skin (~2–3 weeks)
Tdap (tetanus, diphtheria, acellular pertussis for ages 11–64 years) (Adacel®, Boostrix®)	Erythema at injection site	Myalgia, feverish sensation	Allergic reaction to IZ (rare)
Tetanus diphtheria (Td)	Erythema, soreness at injection site	None reported	Allergic reaction to IZ (rare)
Varicella (chickenpox)	Soreness at injection site	Fever, mild rash up to 1 month post-IZ	Seizure, pneumonia
Zoster (shingles, Zostavax®)	Soreness at injection site	Headache (1 in 70)	None reported

Source: www.cdc.gov/vaccines/vac-gen/side-effects.htm

Acute, Febrile, Rash-producing Illness		
Clinical condition with causative agent	**Presentation**	**Comments**
Scarlet fever Agent: *S. pyogenes* (group A beta-hemolytic streptococci)	Scarlatina-form or sandpaper-like rash with exudative pharyngitis, fever, headache, tender, localized anterior cervical lymphadenopathy. Rash usually erupts on day 2 of pharyngitis and often peels a few days later.	Presence of rash does not imply a more severe or serious disease or greater risk of contagion. Treatment: Identical to streptococcal pharyngitis, penicillin as first-line therapy, macrolide (azithro-, clarithro-, erythromycin) only in PCN allergy due to issues of bacterial resistance.
Roseola Agent: Human herpesvirus-6 (HHV-6)	Discrete rosy-pink macular or maculopapular rash lasting hours to 3 days that follows a 3- to 7-day period of fever, often quite high	90% of cases seen in children <2 years Febrile seizures in 10% of children affected. Supportive treatment

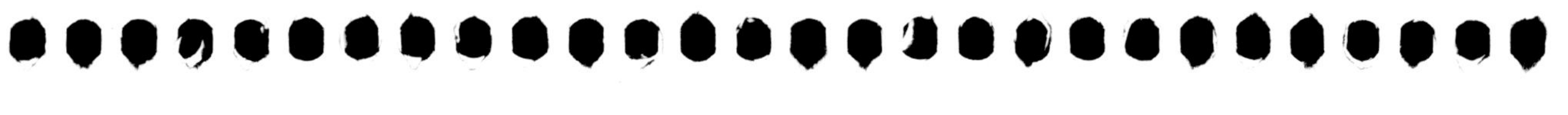

Acute, Febrile, Rash-producing Illness (continued)		
Clinical condition with causative agent	**Presentation**	**Comments**
Rubella Agent: Rubella virus	Mild symptoms; fever, sore throat, malaise, nasal discharge, diffuse maculopapular rash lasting about 3 days Posterior cervical and postauricular lymphadenopathy beginning 5–10 days prior to onset and present during rash Arthralgia in about 25% (most common in women)	Incubation period about 14–21 days with disease transmissible for ~1 week prior to onset of rash to ~2 weeks after rash appears. Generally a mild, self-limiting illness. Greatest risk is effect of virus on the unborn child, especially with first-trimester exposure (~80% rate congenital rubella syndrome). ***Vaccine-preventable disease*** Notifiable disease, usually to the state and/or public health authorities*, laboratory confirmation by presence of serum rubella IgM.

Acute, Febrile, Rash-producing Illness (continued)

Clinical condition with causative agent	Presentation	Comments
Measles Agent: Rubeola virus	Usually acute presentation with fever, nasal discharge, cough, generalized lymphadenopathy, conjunctivitis (copious clear discharge), photophobia, Koplik spots (appearing ~2 days prior to onset of rash as white spots with blue rings held within red spots in oral mucosa) Pharyngitis is usually mild without exudate. Maculopapular rash onset 3–4 days after onset of symptoms, may coalesce to generalized erythema.	Incubation period ~10–14 days with disease transmissible for ~1 week prior to onset of rash to ~2–3 weeks after rash appears. CNS and respiratory tract complications common. Permanent neurologic impairment or death possible. Supportive treatment as well as intervention for complications ***Vaccine-preventable disease*** Notifiable disease, usually to the state and/or public health authorities*, laboratory confirmation by presence of serum rubeola IgM.

Acute, Febrile, Rash-producing Illness (continued)		
Clinical condition with causative agent	**Presentation**	**Comments**
Infectious mononucleosis (IM) Agent: Epstein-Barr virus (human herpesvirus 4)	Maculopapular rash in ~20%, rare petechial rash Fever, "shaggy" purple-white exudative pharyngitis, malaise, marked diffuse lymphadenopathy, hepatic and splenic tenderness with occasional enlargement Diagnostic testing: Heterophil antibody test (Monospot®), leukopenia with lymphocytosis and atypical lymphocytes	Incubation period 20–50 days >90% will develop a rash if given amoxicillin or ampicillin during the illness. Potential for respiratory distress when enlarged tonsils and lymphoid tissue impinges on the upper airway; corticosteroids may be helpful. Splenomegaly most often occurs between days 6 and 21 after onset of illness. Avoid contact sports for ≥1 month due to risk of splenic rupture.
Hand, foot, and mouth disease Agent: Coxsackie virus A16	Fever, malaise, sore mouth, anorexia; 1–2 days later, lesions; also can cause conjunctivitis, pharyngitis Duration of illness: 2–7 days	Transmission via oral-fecal or droplet Highly contagious with incubation period of 2–6 weeks Supportive treatment, analgesia important

Acute, Febrile, Rash-producing Illness (continued)		
Clinical condition with causative agent	**Presentation**	**Comments**
Fifth's disease Agent: Human parvovirus B19	3–4 days of mild, flu-like illness, followed by 7–10 days of red rash that begins on face with "slapped-cheek" appearance, spreads to trunk and extremities. Rash onset corresponds with disease immunity with patient. Viremic and contagious prior to but not after onset of rash.	Droplet transmission; leukopenia common Risk of hydrops fetalis with resulting pregnancy loss when contracted by woman during pregnancy Supportive treatment
Acute HIV infection Agent: Human immunodeficiency virus	Maculopapular rash, fever, mild pharyngitis, ulcerating oral lesions, diarrhea, diffuse lymphadenopathy	Most likely to occur in response to infection with large viral load Consult with HIV specialist concerning initiation of antiretroviral therapy.

Acute, Febrile, Rash-producing Illness (continued)		
Clinical condition with causative agent	**Presentation**	**Comments**
Kawasaki disease Agent: Unknown	For acute-phase illness (usually lasts about 11 days), fever with T≥104°F (40°C) lasting ≥5 days, polymorphic exanthem on trunk, flexor regions, and perineum, erythema of the oral cavity (“strawberry tongue”) with extensively chapped lips, bilateral conjunctivitis, usually without eye discharge, cervical lymphadenopathy, edema and erythema of the hands and feet with peeling skin (late finding, usually 1–2 weeks after onset of fever), no other illness accountable for the findings	Usually in children ages 1–8 years Treatment with IV immunoglobulin and PO aspirin during the acute phase is associated with a reduction in rate of coronary abnormalities, such as coronary artery dilation and coronary aneurysm. Requires expert consultation and treatment advice about accurate diagnosis, aspirin use and ongoing monitoring warranted, usually at a tertiary pediatric medical center.

Source: Fitzgerald, M. A. (2017) Pediatrics, Nurse Practitioner Certification Examination and Practice Preparation, 5th Edition, Philadelphia, PA: F. A. Davis.

***A notifiable disease is one for which regular, frequent, and timely information regarding individual cases is considered necessary for the prevention and control of the disease.* Reference on diseases considered to be notifiable, usually to the state and/or public health authorities is available at website http://www.cdc.gov/mmwr/mmwr_nd/; http://www.cdc.gov/mmwr/volumes/63/wr/mm6354a1.htm?s_cid=mm6354al. Also check with state public health department to receive direction on notification.**

Differential Diagnosis of Wheeze in Children		
Condition	**Features**	**Intervention**
Acute bronchiolitis	Often called the "disease of the happy wheezer," with a mildly ill child, 3 mo–3 y (most age <1 y), viral etiology, most often from respiratory syncytial virus (RSV), less commonly from influenza or adenovirus, short-term acute illness with wheezing often persisting ~3 wk. Most serious in early infancy (<3 mos) and preterm infants. Nearly all episodes occur between November and April.	Supportive, little evidence that inhaled bronchodilators (albuterol, epinephrine) or inhaled or systemic corticosteroids are helpful. Palivizumab (Synagis®) often used to prevent RSV infection in premature infants (first RSV season for infants born at <35 weeks' gestation; infants with chronic lung disease, congenital heart disease, or immune deficiency syndromes).
Acute bronchitis	Viral etiology, short-term, self-limiting	Supportive, perhaps inhaled $beta_2$-agonist, oral anti-inflammatory treatment

Differential Diagnosis of Wheeze in Children (continued)		
Condition	**Features**	**Intervention**
Asthma	Allergic, inflammatory etiology, symptoms recurrent, persistent without treatment	Per NIH Guidelines

Sources: https://pediatrics.aappublications.org/content/134/5/e1474

The American Academy of Pediatrics: Diagnosis and Management of Bronchiolitis: Subcommittee on Diagnosis and Management of Bronchiolitis,

Palivizumab Prophylaxis: https://pediatrics.aappublications.org/content/134/2/e620.full.pdf+html?sid=5002e334-5385-4b37-a30d-97fc7be9a95f

Clinical practice guideline for management of asthma in children and adults, available at http://www.nhlbi.nih.gov/health-pro/guidelines/current/asthma-guidelines

Differential Diagnosis of Stridor in Children

Condition	Features	Intervention
Croup (laryngotracheobronchitis)	Viral, allergic in origin, most common ages 6 months to 5 years	Supportive treatment, perhaps systemic corticosteroid therapy
Foreign body	Acute onset from mechanical obstruction, most common in toddlers	Removal, referral to appropriate care setting such as ED
Congenital obstruction	Present from birth	Surgical repair usually indicated
Peritonsillar abscess	Usually bacterial, most often in older child or adult, usually presents with "hot potato" voice, difficulty swallowing, trismus, contralateral uvula deviation	Attention to airway maintenance, referral to appropriate care setting such as ED, prompt ENT consult, antimicrobial therapy, usually inpatient admission, and perhaps surgical intervention
Acute epiglottitis	Bacterial origin (most often *H. influenzae* type B, potentially preventable with Hib vaccine), most often in children ages 2–7 years. Abrupt onset of high-grade fever, sore throat, dysphagia, and drooling	Attention to airway maintenance, referral to appropriate care setting such as ED, prompt ENT consult, antimicrobial therapy, usually inpatient admission

Source: Stridor, available at emedicine.medscape.com/article/995267-overview

Lactation Risk with Medication Category	
Risk Category	**Examples**
L1- Safest, controlled study= Fail to demonstrate risk	Acetaminophen, penicillins, DMPA (Depo-Provera®) (≥3 weeks post birth)
L2- Safer, limited number of woman studied without risk	Macrolides, nitrofurantoin, cephalosporins, 2d generation antihistamines, prednisone, SSRI
L3- Moderately safe, no controlled study or controlled study shows minimal, non life-threatening risk	TMP-SMX, FQ antibiotics, 1st generation antihistamines, doxycycline
L4- Hazardous, positive evidence of risk, may be used if maternal life-threatening situation	Lithium, ergot preparations, high-dose daily corticosteroids, such as equivalent of prednisone ≥10 mg per day for ≥1 month
L5- Contraindicated, significant and documented risk	Radioactive isotopes, cocaine

Source: Hale, T. (2017) ***Medication and Mother's Milk,*** **17th Edition. New York, NY: Springer Publishing.**

Car Safety Seat Use: The Latest American Academy of Pediatrics Recommendations

Age	Type of seat	General guideline
Infants–age 2 years	Rear-facing	**Rear-facing car seat until 2 years of age** or until the child reaches the highest weight or height allowed by the car safety seat's manufacturer
Toddlers/ preschoolers	Convertible seats and forward-facing seats with harnesses	**All children 2 years or older**, or those younger than 2 years who have outgrown the rear-facing weight or height limit for their car safety seat, should use a **forward-facing car safety seat with a harness for as long as possible**, up to the highest weight or height allowed by their car safety seat's manufacturer.
School-aged children	Booster	All children whose weight or height is above the forward-facing limit for their car safety seat should use a **belt-positioning booster seat** until the vehicle seat belt fits properly, typically when they have reached 4 feet 9 inches (144.8 cm) in height and are between 8 and 12 years of age.

Car Safety Seat Use: The Latest American Academy of Pediatrics Recommendations (continued)		
Age	**Type of seat**	**General guideline**
Older children	Seat belts	When children are old enough and large enough to use the vehicle seat belt alone, they should always use lap and shoulder seat belts for optimal protection. **All children younger than 13 years should be restrained in the rear seats of vehicles for optimal protection.**

Source:

http://pediatrics.aappublications.org/content/early/2011/03/21/peds.2011-0213.full.pdf+html

Micronutrient Requirements for Children		
Nutrient	**Age and daily requirement**	**Comment**
Calcium	Toddler (1–3 years)=500 mg Preschool, younger school age (4–8 years)=800 mg Older children to teens (9–18 years)=1300 mg	1 cup (0.24 L) milk, yogurt=Approximately 250 mg calcium 1 cup (0.24 L) collards, frozen, boiled=357 mg calcium 1 cup (0.24 L) black-eyed peas, boiled=211 mg calcium 3 oz (1/4 block, 85.05 g) calcium-set tofu=163 mg calcium 1 cup (0.24 L) cottage cheese, 1% milk fat=138 mg calcium 1 cup (0.24 L) soy milk=93 mg calcium 1 oz (24 nuts/28.35 g) almonds=70 mg calcium

Micronutrient Requirements for Children (continued)

Nutrient	Age and daily requirement	Comment
Vitamin D	400 IU daily	Difficult to achieve this level with food or with sun exposure that most children experience 1 L of infant formula or vitamin D-fortified cow's milk contains at least 400 IU vitamin D. All non-breastfed infants ingesting <1,000 mL/day of vitamin D-fortified formula or milk should receive a vitamin D supplement of 400 IU/day. AAP recommends that exclusively and partially breastfed infants receive supplements of 400 IU/day of vitamin D shortly after birth and continue to receive these supplements until they are weaned and then consume ≥1,000 mL/day of vitamin D-fortified formula or whole milk. Sun exposure's contribution to vitamin D status is dependent on latitude of residence, skin tone, use of sunscreen, amount of clothing covering the skin, and a number of other factors.

Source: Abrams SA. Dietary Guidelines for Calcium and Vitamin D: A New Era. *Pediatrics*. 2011;127;566. Available at https://pediatrics.aappublications.org/content/127/3/566; Summary of Vitamin D, Calcium, and Iron recommendations available at: https://www.healthychildren.org/English/ages-stages/baby/feeding-nutrition/Pages/Vitamin-Iron-Supplements.aspx

Diagnosis and Prevention of Iron Deficiency and Iron-deficiency Anemia in Infants and Young Children (0–3 Years)
Preterm infants receiving breast milk should receive 2 mg/kg/d of elemental iron through supplements or foods starting by age 1 month through 12 months.
Among preterm infants receiving infant formula, iron supplements could be required, depending on multiple factors influencing iron status.
Term infants taking more than one-half of feedings as human milk should receive 1 mg/kg/d of supplemental iron starting at age 4 months until the introduction of complementary foods (fortified cereals, legumes, red meats, dark green vegetables, vitamin C-containing foods [to enhance iron absorption]).
Term formula-fed infants receive enough iron from formula with the introduction of iron-containing complementary foods after ages 4 to 6 months.
Toddlers can receive adequate iron through heme sources of iron (red meat), nonheme sources (legumes, cereal), and vitamin C-containing foods to promote iron absorption.
Toddlers who do not ingest adequate iron-containing food can receive iron supplements.

Diagnosis and Prevention of Iron Deficiency and Iron-deficiency Anemia in Infants and Young Children (0–3 Years) (continued)

In treating an infant, child, or adult with established iron-deficiency anemia (IDA), supplemental iron should be continued for about 2 months after correction of the anemia and its etiologic cause in order to replenish body stores of iron.

- Ongoing evaluation for iron deficiency is an important part of providing primary care for the young child. All children should be screened for IDA through hemoglobin measurement at age 1 year.
    - With Hb<10 g/dL, further testing to confirm iron deficiency, such as ferritin
    - With milder anemia (Hb 10–11 g/dL), an alternative evaluation plan includes treating with iron for 1 month. A rise in Hb ≥1 g/dL after a month of iron therapy helps to confirm iron deficiency, particularly if additional clinical assessment helps to support the diagnosis.

Source: Clinical report—diagnosis and prevention of iron deficiency and iron-deficiency anemia in infants and young children (0–3 years of age), available at http://pediatrics.aappublications.org/content/early/2010/10/05/peds.2010-2576.full.pdf+html

Helpful Numbers	
Poison control	**1-800-222-1222** www.safekids.org/safety-basics/safety-guide/medication-safety-guide/find-a-poison-control-center.html?gclid=CLTQmeqamLMCFREx4AodeHAAhQ
Seat check	**1-866-732-8243**

Helpful Guidelines	
American Academy of Pediatric Dentistry	www.aapd.org
Centers for Disease Control and Prevention, Consumer Product Safety Commission, and U.S. Fire Administration	www.firesafetyforkids.org
Department of Health and Human Services, National Institute of Health, National Heart Lung and Blood Institute People Science Health; Blood Pressure tables	www.nhlbi.nih.gov/health-pro/guidelines/current/hypertension-pediatric-jnc-4/blood-pressure-tables
U.S. Environmental Protection Agency	www.epa.gov

XX. Resources and Guidelines

Recommendations for Preventive Pediatric Health Care	
Advisory Committee on Immunization Practices (ACIP)	www.cdc.gov/vaccines
American Academy of Pediatrics, Car Seat Safety	www.healthychildren.org/English/safety-prevention/on-the-go/Pages/Car-Safety-Seats-Information-for-Families.aspx
American Academy of Pediatrics, Red Book Online	redbook.solutions.aap.org/redbook.aspx
American Academy of Otolaryngology – Head and Neck Surgery – Clinical Practice Guidelines	www.entnet.org/content/clinical-practice-guidelines
American Heart Association	www.heart.org/HEARTORG/
BMI Calculator CDC Growth Charts: United States	www.cdc.gov/growthcharts/
Bright Futures	brightfutures.org/

Recommendations for Preventive Pediatric Health Care (continued)	
Bright Futures in Practice: Mental Health—Volume II, Tool Kit Tools for Health Professionals	www.brightfutures.org/mentalhealth/pdf/tools.html
Center for Disease Control and Prevention	www.cdc.gov
Department of Human and Health Services, Morbidity and Mortality Weekly	www.cdc.gov/mmwr
AAP Developmental and Behavioral Pediatrics	www2.aap.org/sections/dbpeds/
KySS℠ Guide to Child and Adolescent Mental Health Screening, Early Intervention and Health Promotion	www.napnap.org/mental-health-guide
Lead Home/Lead Awareness Program	www2.epa.gov/lead
March of Dimes	www.marchofdimes.org/
Maternal and Child Health Library	www.ncbi.nlm.nih.gov/pmc/articles/PMC314116/

Recommendations for Preventive Pediatric Health Care (continued)	
NAPNAP's PNP Position Statements	www.napnap.org/napnap-position-statements-0
National Highway Traffic Safety Administration	www.nhtsa.dot.gov
Treating Tobacco Use and Dependence AHRQ	www.ahrq.gov/professionals/clinicians-providers/guidelines-recommendations/tobacco/index.html
Patient Healthcare Questionnaires Screeners, Pfizer, Inc.	www.phqscreeners.com
U.S. Department of Agriculture Mypyramid	www.choosemyplate.gov/

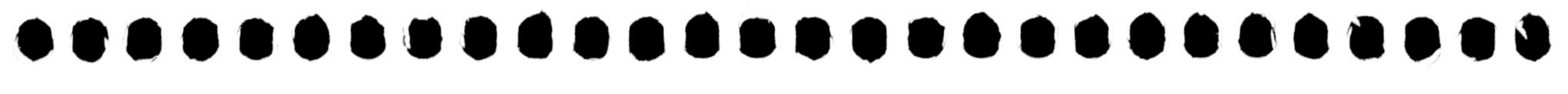

Recommendations for Preventive Pediatric Health Care (continued)	
U.S. Preventive Services Task Force (USPSTF) Guide to Clinical Preventive Services, Department of Health and Human Services, Agency for Healthcare Research and Quality	www.ahrq.gov/professionals/clinicians-providers/guidelines-recommendations/uspstf/index.html
U.S. Surgeon General's Family History Initiative	www.hhs.gov/familyhistory

Resources for Additional Study

Books:

Fitzgerald, M. A. (2017) Pediatrics, in Study Guide for Family Nurse Practitioner Certification Examination and Practice Preparation, 5th Edition, Philadelphia, PA: F. A. Davis.

Audio programs:

Fitzgerald, M. A. Bacterial Pharyngitis, Conjunctivitis, Acute Otitis Media: A Focus on Latest Treatment Recommendations, North Andover, MA: Fitzgerald Health Education Associates, LLC

Miller, S. K. Prescribing for the Relief of Symptoms, North Andover, MA: Fitzgerald Health Education Associates, LLC

Yates, C.M. Asthma Update: An Evidence-based Approach to Management throughout the Lifespan, North Andover, MA: Fitzgerald Health Education Associates, LLC

Yates, C.M. Acute Asthma Exacerbations and Acute Uncomplicated Bronchitis: An Evidence-based Approach to Management, North Andover, MA: Fitzgerald Health Education Associates, LLC

References

Allen, P.J., Vessey, J.A., & Schapiro, N. (2010). *Primary Care of the Child with a Chronic Condition*. 5th Edition. St. Louis, MO: Mosby/Elsevier.

Burns, C.E., Dunn, A.M., Brady, M.A., Starr, N.B., & Blosser, C.G. (2017). *Pediatric Primary Care*. 6h Edition. St. Louis, MO: Saunders/Elsevier.

Daniels, S.R. & Greer, F.R. (2008) Committee on Nutrition Lipid Screening and Cardiovascular Health in Childhood. *Pediatrics, 122 (1),* 198–208.

Drotar, D., Stancin, T., Dworkin, P.H., Sices, L. & Wood, S. (2008) Selecting Developmental Surveillance and Screening Tools. *Pediatrics in Review*, 2008; 29:52–58.

Duderstadt, K. (2013). *Pediatric Physical Examination: An Illustrated Handbook*, 2nd Edition. St. Louis, MO: Elsevier/Mosby.

Hagan, J.F., Shaw, J.S., & Duncan, P.M. Eds. (2008). *Bright Futures: Guidelines for Health Supervision of Infants, Children, and Adolescents*, 3rd Edition. Elk Grove Village, IL: American Academy of Pediatrics.

Johnson, R.A. & Wolff, K. (2013). *Fitzpatrick's Color Atlas and Synopsis of Clinical Dermatology*, 7th Edition, New York, NY: McGraw Hill.

Kleinman, R.E. Ed. (2014). *Pediatric Nutrition Handbook,* 7th Edition. Elk Grove Village, IL: American Academy of Pediatrics.

McCance, K. (2014). *Pathophysiology: The Biologic basis for disease in Adults and Children,* 7th Edition, St. Louis, MO: Elsevier.

NONPF Core Competencies available at http://www.nonpf.org/?page=14

Rice, S.G and the Council on Sports Medicine and Fitness (2008). Medical conditions affecting sports participation. *Pediatrics, 121 (4),* 841–848.

Silbert-Flagg, J. (2017) *Pediatric Nurse Practitioner Certification Review Guide: Primary Care*, 6th Edition, Sudbury, MA: Jones & Bartlett Publishers.

Silbert-Flagg, J. (2011) *Pediatric Nurse Practitioner Certification Study Question Book*, 3rd Edition, Sudbury, MA: Jones & Bartlett Publishers.

USDHHS. *Guide to Clinical Preventive Services, Recommendations of the U.S. Preventive Services Task Force https://www.uspreventiveservicestaskforce.org/Announcements/News/Item/uspstf-releases-2014-guide-to-clinical-preventive-services*

All website addresses and phone numbers cited in this document were active when published. Many are sources created and maintained by organizations other than FHEA; in these instances, the websites are subject to change over time and out of our control.